12th Workshop Conference Hoechst

THE IMPORTANCE OF ISLETS OF LANGERHANS FOR MODERN ENDOCRINOLOGY

12th Workshop Conference Hoechst
Schloss Reisensburg
April 16–18, 1982

The Importance of Islets of Langerhans for Modern Endocrinology

Editors

Konrad F. Federlin, M.D.
Professor of Internal Medicine
III Medical Clinic and
Policlinic
University of Giessen
Giessen, F.R.G.

Josef Scholtholt, M.D.
Honorary Professor of
Physiology
University of Frankfurt
Hoechst AG
Frankfurt, F.R.G.

Raven Press New York

Raven Press, 1140 Avenue of the Americas, New York, New York 10036

© 1984 by Raven Press Books, Ltd. All rights reserved. This book is protected by copyright. No part of it may be reproduced, stored in a retrieval system, or transmitted, in any form or by any means, electronic, mechanical, photocopying, recording, or otherwise, without the prior written permission of the publisher.

Made in the United States of America

Library of Congress Cataloging in Publication Data

Workshop Conference Hoechst (12th : 1982 : Schloss Reisenburg)
   The importance of islets of Langerhans for modern endocrinology.

   Hoechst workshop series)
   Includes bibliographies and index.
   1. Diabetes—Congresses.   2. Islands of Langerhans—Congresses.   I. Federlin, Konrad F.   II. Scholtholt, Josef.   III. Title.   IV. Series. [DNLM: 1. Islands of Langerhans—Congresses.   2. Diabetes mellitus—Congresses. W3 WO51M 12th 1982i / WK 800 W926 1982i]
   RC660.A15W66   1982   616.4'62   82-04251
   ISBN 0-89004-939-4

   The material contained in this volume was submitted as previously unpublished material, except in the instances in which credit has been given to the source from which some of the illustrative material was derived.
   Great care has been taken to maintain the accuracy of the information contained in the volume. However, Raven Press cannot be held responsible for errors or for any consequences arising from the use of the information contained herein.

Preface

Many years have passed since the first histological description of the islets of Langerhans, leading to the discovery of the importance of the pancreas for diabetes, the isolation of insulin, and the beginnings of our understanding of the molecular mechanisms of the interaction between insulin and its receptors. The geographical distribution of different cellular components of the islets of Langerhans, either within the islets themselves or within the pancreas, is an indication of the complex endocrine function of the organ. The somewhat singular view of the pancreas has changed and the total gastrointestinal system has been recognized as a very complex endocrine organ which is receiving increasing attention.

This volume presents past and future research aspects of the gastrointestinal endocrine system with emphasis toward the importance of the islets of Langerhans for diabetes mellitus. It will be of interest for endocrinologists, biochemists, pharmacologists, diabetologists, and physicians in general who deal with the daily problem of diabetes mellitus and its different treatment possibilities.

J. Scholtholt

Contents

1 Opening Address
K. F. Federlin

11 Cellular Relationships in the Islet of Langerhans: A Regulatory Perspective
L. Orci

27 Evidence of a Glucose-Sensitive Process in the Beta Cell that Regulates Preferential Secretion of Newly Synthesized Insulin
Gerold M. Grodsky, Gerald Gold, Herbert D. Landahl, Mikhail L. Gishizky, and Robert E. Nowlain

41 Subunit Structures and Actions of the Receptors for Insulin and the Insulin-like Growth Factors
Michael P. Czech, Joan Massague, Kin Yu, Catherine L. Oppenheimer, and Cristina Mottola

55 Gastrointestinal Hormones and Islet Function
Werner Creutzfeldt

69 Insulin-like Growth Factors and Somatomedin
H. Ditschuneit and B. Pfeifle

93 Pathomorphology of the Pancreas in Diabetes
W. Gepts

111 Diabetes and Virus
Horst Müntefering

129 Treatment of Diabetes Mellitus: Oral Hypoglycemic Agents
Sotirios Raptis

165 Treatment of Diabetes Mellitus: Insulin
Karl Schöffling, Christoph Rosak, and Peter-Henning Althoff

189 Artificial Endocrine Pancreas and Portable Insulin Pumps: Effect of Improved Glucose Control on Hor-

monal and Metabolic Abnormalities and the Development of Microvascular Complications in Type I Diabetes
Wolfgang Kerner

205 Pancreas-Islet Transplantation
K. F. Federlin and R. G. Bretzel

225 Afterword
Rachmiel Levine

231 Subject Index

Contributors

Peter-Henning Althoff
Department of Endocrinology
and Metabolism
Center of Internal Medicine
Johann Wolfgang Goethe
University
D-6000 Frankfurt am Main
Federal Republic of Germany

R. G. Bretzel
III Medical Clinic and
Polyclinic
University of Giessen
D-6300 Giessen, Federal
Republic of Germany

Werner Creutzfeldt
Medical Clinic and Policlinic
Clinics of the University of
Göttingen
D-3400 Göttingen, Federal
Republic of Germany

Michael P. Czech
Department of Biochemistry
University of Massachusetts
Medical Center
Worcester, Massachusetts
01605

H. Ditschuneit
Department of Internal
Medicine II
University of Ulm
D-7900 Ulm, Federal Republic
of Germany

Konrad F. Federlin
Professor of Internal Medicine
III Medical Clinic and Policlinic
University of Giessen
D-6300 Giessen, Federal
Republic of Germany

W. Gepts
Department of Pathology
Fak. Geneeskunde & Farmacie
Vrije Universiteit Brussel
B-7090 Brussels, Belgium

Mikhail L. Gishizky
Metabolic Research Unit and
Department of Biochemistry
and Biophysics
University of California at San
Francisco
San Francisco, California
94143

Gerald Gold
Metabolic Research Unit and
Department of Biochemistry
and Biophysics
University of California at San
Francisco
San Francisco, California
94143

Gerold M. Grodsky
Metabolic Research Unit and
Department of Biochemistry
and Biophysics
University of California at San
Francisco
San Francisco, California
94143

CONTRIBUTORS

Wolfgang Kerner
Department of Internal
 Medicine I
University of Ulm
D 7900 Ulm, Federal Republic
 of Germany

Herbert D. Landahl
Metabolic Research Unit and
 Department of Biochemistry
University of California at San
 Francisco
San Francisco, California
 94143

Rachmiel Levine
City of Hope Medical Center
Duarte, California 91010

Joan Massague
Department of Biochemistry
University of Massachusetts
 Medical Center
Worcester, Massachusetts
 01605

Cristina Mottola
Department of Biochemistry
University of Massachusetts
 Medical Center
Worcester, Massachusetts
 01605

Horst Müntefering
Department of Pediatric
 Pathology
Institute of Pathology
Johannes Gutenberg University
6500 Mainz, Federal Republic
 of Germany

Robert E. Nowlain
Metabolic Research Unit and
 Department of Biochemistry
 and Biophysics
University of California at San
 Francisco 94143
San Francisco, California
 94143

Catherine L. Oppenheimer
Department of Biochemistry
University of Massachusetts
 Medical Center
Worcester, Massachusetts
 01605

L. Orci
Institute of Histology and
 Embryology
University of Geneva Medical
 School
Geneva, Switzerland

B. Pfeifle
Department of Internal
 Medicine II
University of Ulm 7900 Ulm,
 Federal Republic of
 Germany

Sotorios Raptis
Department of Internal
 Medicine
Evangelismos Hospital
Athens University
Athens, Greece

Christoph Rosak
Department of Endocrinology
 and Metabolism
Center of Internal Medicine
Johann Wolfgang Goethe
 University
D-6000 Frankfurt am Main,
 Federal Republic of Germany

Karl Schöffling
Department of Endocrinology
 and Metabolism

Center of Internal Medicine
Johann Wolfgang Goethe
 University
D-6000 Frankfurt am Main,
 Federal Republic of Germany

Josef Scholtholt
Honorary Professor of
 Physiology
University of Frankfurt

Hoechst AG
Frankfurt, Federal Republic
 of Germany

Kin Yu
Department of Biochemistry
University of Massachusetts
 Medical Center
Worcester, Massachusetts
 01605

12th Workshop Conference Hoechst

THE IMPORTANCE OF ISLETS OF LANGERHANS FOR MODERN ENDOCRINOLOGY

Opening Address

Konrad F. Federlin

Medical Clinic and Policlinic III, University of Giessen, Giessen, Federal Republic of Germany

It is my privilege to extend, also on behalf of Professor Scholtholt from Hoechst AG, a warm welcome to you who have come to this scientific symposium held in honor of Professor Dr. h.c. Ernst-Friedrich Pfeiffer on the occasion of his 60th birthday. It was the wish of Dr. Pfeiffer that these scientific lectures emphasize the importance of the islets of Langerhans for modern endocrinology. This would not be possible without the contribution of many renowned international and national researchers in the field of experimental and clinical medicine. They are the ones I would like to thank first and foremost, not only on Professor Pfeiffer's behalf but also on my own. The inclusion of their articles depicting the present state of accomplishments in their individual fields of research is a valuable gift to Professor Pfeiffer as well as to the scientific community.

Our special thanks to Hoechst AG, and particularly its representatives, Professor von Wasielewski and Professor Scholtholt. Connections between the 60th birthday of Professor Pfeiffer and a company that is outside the Federal Republic of Germany, one of the leading firms engaged worldwide in finding new ways of treating diabetes mellitus—in additional to many years of cooperation ranging from sulfonylurea to the artificial pancreas—speak for themselves. The representatives of this company not only organized the symposium on which this volume is based, but also provided the framework that facilitated the meeting in the first place. Without Professor Scholtholt and the active support and assistance of his secretariat, we would not have been able to realize our plans.

Let me now return to the person and the topic of focus in this book: Ernst Pfeiffer and the islets of Langerhans. Could there be a better metaphor for describing efforts in science to obtain medical and natural scientific knowledge than the exploration of a mysterious, unknown island? Situated in the ocean of nescience for thousands of years and eventually discovered by the German pathologist Paul Langerhans in the last century, it still is the fascinating destination of innumerable scientists all over the world. Some of the scientific explorers go ashore left entirely to their own devices—with rucksack and hiking boots, so to speak—to wheedle a secret out of the island, whereas others arrive as a well-equipped expedition with numerous bearers and several Biostators® in their baggage train. Under the guidance of an experienced explorer, they venture to the center of the island where, in the jungle of beta, alpha, delta, and pp cells, hindered by the network of capillary rivers, harried by antibodies and lymphocytes, and led astray by false hypotheses, they try to find the scientific treasure and make their scientific fortune.

We have come together to honor one of the most renowned explorers of this island today, and although without any doubt, his 60th birthday will not retire his march to the central parts of the island, but provides a moment that we may reflect on his personal and professional itinerary.

Ernst Pfeiffer, the leader of our expedition, was born in 1922, which means that he came into this world in a rather turbulent year. Let us recall: in 1922 The Soviet Union was founded; Mussolini assumed power in Italy; a huge wave of terrorism, culminating in the assassination of Walter Rathenau, swept over Germany; a disarmament conference was held in Washington; Berlin became a cultural center of worldwide reputation; Wilhelm Furtwängler started his career as orchestra conductor; Arnold Schönberg introduced twelve-tone music; and Alfredo Cordona performed a triple somersault from trapeze to trapeze, according to Stein's cultural almanac. But 1922 was also the year in which the first long-term study of diabetes treatment with the hormone insulin, discovered in the previous year, was published.

If the year of Ernst Pfeiffer's birth was turbulent, the following years were hardly less so: inflation, worldwide economic crisis and then Hitler's seizure of power with its devastating consequences for the world and for Germany. Drafted in 1941, Ernst Pfeiffer was of the age group that suffered the most severe decimation, yet he survived 4 years of war and ventured into a new, uncertain life amidst the rubble of his country. Ernst Pfeiffer's experiences and contacts, in war and captivity, repeatedly influenced the course of his life. For example, the British military hospital in Italy, to which he was brought as a prisoner of war, treated even German wounded soldiers with penicillin for the first time in history. This was an incident that turned out to be a stroke of luck for an unproblematic doctoral thesis back in Germany a few years later. Also, it seems paradigmatic that in this British unit the young German junior physician had already met a Major Sheehan, who would very soon become renowned worldwide by the medical profession as the first physician to describe an important syndrome in endocrinology.

Having begun his medical studies in Munich during the war, Ernst Pfeiffer continued his studies in Heidelberg and completed them in 1948 in Frankfurt. Prior to his graduation, during the war, a meeting of decisive importance took place which has influenced his entire life up to this day. He met a female student in Munich, Margret, who became his life's companion shortly afterward. At the beginning of his internship in Frankfurt, then a medical assistant, Pfeiffer met the great internal specialist Professor Franz Volhard, a man who was and still is his model. During the Third Reich, Professor Volhard had to retire prematurely on the grounds of his antiNazi attitude. After the war, he experienced the satisfaction of heading his former hospital again in the late years of his life. Stories centered around this baroque personality with his many strengths and also weaknesses are legion. The core of this great physician and academic teacher was a high intelligence and extensive knowledge, paired with a particularly pronounced ability to summarize commonplace observations and to synthesize them into an edifice of logical thoughts. Up to this day, i.e., beyond the period of his activity, Professor Volhard has influenced nephrology worldwide. Ernst Pfeiffer, siding his dynamics with the still remarkable activity of his aging clinical teacher, ventured into the first major scientific task transferred to him by Professor Volhard: the pathogenesis of chronic glomerulonephritis. In toilsome clinical trials, using relatively simple biochemical methods, such as the colloid particle method, for complement determination in the serum of patients with an acute or chronic kidney disease on the one hand, or in the artificially induced glomerulonephritis in experimental animals on the other, Pfeiffer tried to do justice to this great task, with support from his early road companion Karl Schöffling and assistance from a large number of co-workers. It was only a few years until, on the basis of parabiotic tests, the hypothesis of a cell-linked immune reaction as the cause of chronicity in experimentally induced glomerulonephritis was developed. With the habilitation thesis that he submitted in 1954, Pfeiffer drew a first concluding stroke under this work that, unfortunately, Franz Volhard did not live to see.

Another great yet completely different clinician, Ferdinand Hoff, had been assigned as the director of the I. Medizinische Universitätsklinik in 1951 in Frankfurt. Like all of those who were fortunate enough to work and learn under the aegis of this outstanding physician, young docent Pfeiffer, who soon was appointed senior physician, owed essential impulses to him, among them the ones concerning the endocrine system, and thus a course in research that is followed up to this day.

Ernst Pfeiffer returned from a postgraduate Fulbright scholarship in the United States in 1957–1958 with a host of new ideas for further research activities in the field of experiment-induced glomerulonephritis. The transatlantic transfer of the method of immunofluorescence, which he had learned from Albert Coons, the old master himself, and the new knowledge on kidney immunology and transplantation, which he had picked up from John Merrill at Harvard University, spurred on the working team around Ernst Pfeiffer, which had by no means been idle in previous years, to even greater vigor. Each doctoral candidate available, who was familiar with the technique of inducing Masugi-glomerulonephritis and with the technique of parabiosis, i.e., the side-to-side union of two animals for the purpose of developing a blood-tissue bridge, worked in one of the many individual research groups under the supervision of experienced laboratory assistants. Under still rather primitive conditions—each empty room of the hospital was converted into a provisional Pfeiffer laboratory—and with an enthusiasm hardly imaginable today, this huge team worked after duty hours until midnight and even later, including weekends, urged on by nothing but the air of activity emanating from Ernst Pfeiffer and an interest in the new and unknown. The highlight of these activities was the congress of internal specialists held in Wiesbaden 20 years ago, where Professor Hoff, our honored head of the clinic, held the chair, and where kidney immunology, one of the focal topics of the congress, became a point of controversy between the group around Professor Sarre from Freiburg and our group from Frankfurt. The issue in question was whether autoimmunity was the cause of chronicity in glomerulonephritis, which we felt we had proved, or whether other, still unknown factors were responsible for the chronicity, an opinion which experiments by Professor Sarre's group seemed to prove. Although for many of those present this battle of words may have ended in a draw, findings on the actual participation of autologous kidney antigens in the continuity of chronic glomerulonephritis that were obtained later on, some of them only in recent years, provided a satisfactory, if late, justification for Ernst Pfeiffer, the leader in this battle.

However, around the same time, in the early 1960s, the change in the goals of activity in immunology and endocrinology was in the offing. Markedly influenced by his stay with Joslin and Thorn, the leading American endocrinologists at Harvard, Ernst Pfeiffer concentrated more on endocrinology, a field that had been worked on in clinical practice for many years but had only just begun to receive greater scientific attention. With his colleagues Schöffling, Ditschuneit, Retiene, and Melani, Ernst Pfeiffer developed biological methods for measuring ACTH, insulin, and glucagon. Before that, the theory of insulin stimulation in the mechanism of action of sulfonylurea oral antidiabetics had been proved by combined functional biochemical and morphological studies in calves, dogs, and rats. Clearly recognizing the large problems that, at least then, prevented the adoption of immunological methods in clinical medicine, he abandoned immunology and research on kidneys even though he was offered a full professorship at New York Medical College. After his refusal, Ernst Pfeiffer was appointed *extra ordinarius* professor of endocrinology at the I. Medizinische Klinik in Frankfurt. Consequently, endocrinology and particularly the islets of Langerhans became the focus of his scientific interest. Very soon, research on the relationship between gastrointestinal and hypothalamic hormones and the endocrine pancreas was started, and the number of doctoral candidates in this field continued to grow. In animal laboratories of Frankfurt University, originally built for the entire medical faculty but in practice used only by Pfeiffer and his group, up to 80 persons, including all scientific colleagues, laboratory technicians, and doctoral candidates, would meet Wednesday afternoons for the endocrinological seminar. The call to a full professorship of internal medicine at the newly founded University of Ulm and the consequent move of the entire working group, which resembled an exodus from Frankfurt, provided the basis for a fruitful expansion of scientific work. The Ulm concept of establishing focuses in scientific research not only in the field of internal medicine but also in the neighboring disciplines of pediatrics and gynecology, as well as in the theoretical subjects anatomy and biochemistry with scientists active in these fields, provided the opportunity to widen and deepen experimental and clinical research. Despite a certain reduction in the intensity of work during his rectorship from 1975–1979, Pfeiffer's team continued to be one of the most active German groups working in the field of endocrinology. Therefore, the previously started work on the future development of an artificial pancreas was continued and completed in the form of the Biostator®. In spite of the enormous burden as head of the university's administrative body, this position allowed him to realize further plans for the development of internal medicine in Ulm.

If the growth of the working group under the supervision of Ernst Pfeiffer between 1955 and 1965 up to the move to Ulm was phenomenal, its continuous successful regeneration was equally impressive. First, Professor Schöffling left the clinic in Ulm with a large group of young committed assistants and returned to

Frankfurt. Professor Ditschuneit began to concentrate on the related but independent field of fat metabolism, and in the mid-1970s, Professor Raptis, Professor Ziegler, and I embarked to new shores with a large number of assistants.

In terms of the metaphor of the expedition to the island, some experienced scouts may have been lost, but the team continued to recruit new and committed young assistants who gradually replaced those who left. Yet with very few exceptions, the contact with those who had left never broke off, and therefore this retrospect among so many former fellow explorers in this volume may fill the leader of our expedition with joy and satisfaction. It goes without saying that, because of the different characters and temperaments, the years in which we worked together were not devoid of tensions and disputes. The "boss" would become rather impatient and angry if the pace of the many bearers slowed down in the jungle of the island; but up to this day, everyone of them picked up their load again after the storm had blown over, since they felt that the arduous way would finally lead to a rewarding goal.

Now to describe the scientific yield that Ernst Pfeiffer produced in the many years of active research. His achievements found their expression in more than 300 original publications, numerous monographs, and chapters of various books, and especially in the standard work of diabetologists of the last decade, the *Manual of Diabetes mellitus*. They attracted attention at home and abroad and are the basis for numerous honors, such as the chairmanship of the German and European Diabetes Association and of the International Society of Internal Medicine, honorary memberships in many international scientific societies and, as academic highlights, the conferment of the degree of honorary doctor by the Universities of Athens and Cairo.

At the same time, various other associations and groups availed themselves of Ernst Pfeiffer's expert knowledge. To name just a few in representation for many others, let me mention the membership in the foundation committee of the Universities of Ulm and Regensburg, his consultancy in numerous national and international scientific journals, and mainly the foundation and editorship of the renowned journal *Hormone and Metabolic Research*. Although the editorial work and its big resonance among experts alone suffice to qualify Ernst Pfeiffer as a successful scientist, there are also essential aspects of his personality that contributed to his success. I wish to offer a laudation for his deeply satisfying and fulfilling life's work, which doubtlessly required even more than his own application and effort. In returning to the metaphor we should ask how the expedition to the islets of Langerhans was able to get so far under his guidance. Certainly not without an enviably good physical condition which up to this day has permitted him to cope with nightlong work and strenuous travel, often in extremely short intervals. For the most part his shrewd policy, combined with a feeling for upcoming and promising objectives and a clear vision as to which of yesterday's projects were no longer relevant, that caused him to act at the most appropriate times amidst an almost impenetrable thicket of scientific opinions. The gift of reasoning in a manner that convinces and persuades others in favor of his ideas was and is one of Ernst Pfeiffer's qualities essential to his success as a politician. His ability to raise funds for continuous research is no less pronounced. Relying on either the many years of support by the German Research Association for individual or large-scale projects in the field of special research, or on third-party funds, the researchers in Professor Pfeiffer's team always knew that carrying out an envisaged scientific project would *not* fail for lack of financial means. The European and International Diabetes Association also makes very good use of this ability of its treasurer, Dr. Pfeiffer.

Success is guaranteed when the politician and financier complement each other as a good manager, an additional quality of the head of the clinic and sometime dean and rector, Ernst Pfeiffer. Many persons with fine reputations for skillfully delegating work found their master in Pfeiffer. I remember an American colleague who told me that it was not until Pfeiffer had left that he realized he had basically been working more in the interest of his German guest rather than in his own.

Many managers suffer from a sign that not infrequently becomes their undoing: restlessness. In contrast, Ernst Pfeiffer has developed the art of temporarily freeing himself from the pressures of everyday life with its numerous tasks, duties, and commitments by going fishing in the waters around Ulm or by sailing in his boat. When we add the pleasure of travelling, the ability to enjoy culinary delights, and the interest in historical and political literature to this attempted portrait, the picture does not show an austere, withdrawn, or ascetic scientist of the traditional Prussian variety, but rather a lively cosmopolitan professor, a rare species in Germany, who might run a clinic or a university as well as a company, or head a ministry.

Thus, it is the portrait of an *active* man in the sense of our great fellow citizen from Frankfurt that I have tried to outline, the picture of a homo faber, to whom the phrase that in the long run only the hardworking are lucky applies in a particularly large degree. But we must not see all this one-sidedly, without his always sympathetic wife and children, i.e., the family which, in a harmony that has become relatively rare, was and is the basis for his professional activities.

We are nearing the end of the expedition to the islets of Langerhans mentioned at the beginning. The following topics urge us to proceed. Each chapter in this volume is a birthday present for Ernst Pfeiffer, as well as an expression of congratulations, affection, and gratitude.

In an article on the year 1922 recently published in the *Frankfurter Allgemeine Zeitung*, the author, Jürgen Eick, closes with the words, "The only way to live long is to grow old" as a consolation for hardships possibly connected with this year. I would like to counter this wording, which expresses a certain amount of resignation, with the variant, "A successful way to live long is to be as young at the age of 60 as Ernst Pfeiffer."

Cellular Relationships in the Islet of Langerhans: A Regulatory Perspective

L. Orci

Institute of Histology and Embryology, University of Geneva Medical School, Geneva, Switzerland

In this chapter, we will examine some structural features of the islet of Langerhans that are possibly endowed with regulatory influences on islet secretion.

DISTRIBUTION OF ISLET CELLS

Until 1976, the prevalent concept was that the endocrine pancreas consisted of a unique type of islet of Langerhans containing insulin cells, glucagon cells, and a small number of somatostatin and pancreatic-polypeptide-secreting cells. The systematic application of immunocytochemistry to carefully identified pancreatic samples has revealed a more complex situation in both the rodent and human pancreas. When one applies to successive serial sections of the rat pancreas antisera against insulin, glucagon, somatostatin and pancreatic polypeptide, each revealed by the indirect immunofluorescence technique (1), the insulin immunofluorescent cells are seen to form the bulk of the islet where they occupy a central position, whereas glucagon immunofluorescence appears as a rim surrounding the insulin cells; somatostatin cells are also peripheral, as are pancreatic polypeptide-containing cells, although the latter appear much less numerous (Fig. 1). However, as shown in Fig. 2, other islets can be observed in which the number of pancreatic polypeptide cells is high, whereas that of glucagon cells is low; otherwise, such islets reveal proportions of insulin and somatostatin cells approximately similar to those of glucagon-rich

12   CELLULAR RELATIONSHIPS

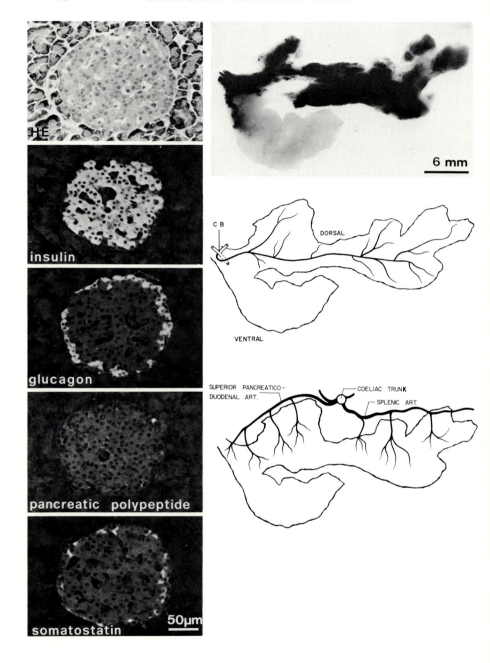

islets. Systematic sampling of islets in various regions of the rat pancreas revealed that glucagon-rich islets came invariably from the tail, body, or superior part of the head of the pancreas (these regions are also called collectively the "dorsal" or "splenic" part of the pancreas), whereas pancreatic-polypeptide-rich islets were always restricted to the middle and inferior part of the head (also called "ventral" or "duodenal" pancreatic region) (2). When this anatomical distribution is related to pancreatic vascularization and exocrine drainage, a nonrandom situation is also evident: glucagon-rich islets belong to the region of the pancreas vascularized by the coeliac trunk via the gastroduodenal and splenic arteries and drained by the main dorsal exocrine duct (see Fig. 1), whereas pancreatic-polypeptide-rich islets are distributed in the pancreatic territories vascularized by the superior mesenteric artery via the inferior pancreaticoduodenal artery and drained by the main ventral (or "distal") exocrine duct (see Fig. 2) (the main dorsal or proximal duct opens separately from the main ventral duct in the bile canal and this separate opening renders possible the retrograde injection of the two tributary territories from which each islet type can be isolated separately) (3,4). Lucite models of the two rat islet types have now been constructed on the basis of serial section reconstruction (Fig. 3), and we can determine the respective numbers and proportions of each endocrine cell type in one of each islet (4, 5).

←───

FIG. 1. Left: Five successive serial sections of an islet from the dorsal part of the pancreas of the rat, stained with hemalum-eosin (HE), and with insulin, glucagon, pancreatic polypeptide and somatostatin antisera, respectively. Note that the homogeneous islet cell mass in HE-stained section appears organized into specific patterns when revealed by the different antisera. In the dorsal type islet, the rim of peripheral cells surrounding the central insulin cell core contains numerous glucagon cells, but very scarce pancreatic polypeptide cells. Somatostatin cells are in intermediate numbers. × 160. **Right:** The *upper panel* represents a rat pancreas *in toto* injected with India ink through the dorsal duct (drawn in *middle panel*). The region blackened by this procedure contains all dorsal-type islets as shown in the left. The *lower panel* illustrates the vascularization of this region. CB = bile canal. × 2.0. (From Orci, ref. 33, with permission).

14 CELLULAR RELATIONSHIPS

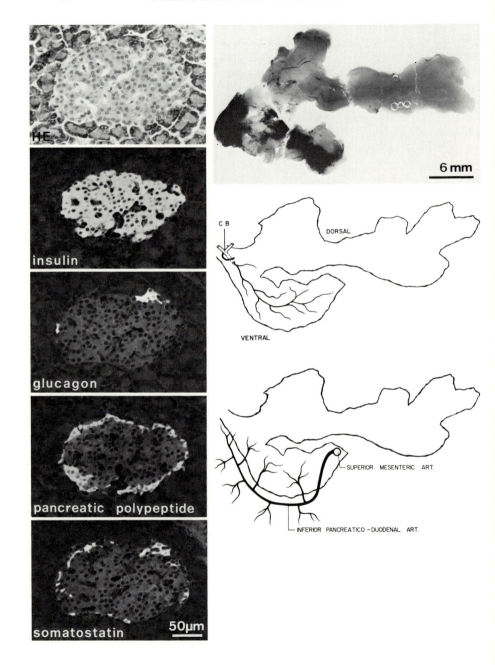

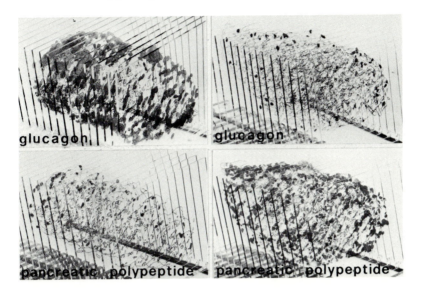

FIG. 3. Lucite model of a dorsal-type (*left*) and ventral-type (*right*) rat pancreatic islet following complete serial sectioning. The Lucite sheets showing the glucagon and pancreatic polypeptide cells have been mounted. The dark spots represent individual cells and this emphasizes their reverse proportion in each islet. The dorsal islet represented here had a total of 3,126 endocrine cells from which 2,063 were insulin cells, 874 glucagon cells, 66 pancreatic-polypeptide cells and 123 somatostatin cells. The ventral islet shown had a total of 4,136 cells with 3,061 insulin cells, 67 glucagon cells, 818 pancreatic-polypeptide cells and 190 somatostatin cells. (From Baetens et. al., ref. 3; Orci and Perrelet, refs. 4 and 5; with permission).

FIG. 2. Left and right: Same experimental design as described in Fig. 1, but from a ventral-type islet. Note the abundance of pancreatic polypeptide cells in the peripheral rim and the sparsity of glucagon cells in such islets; the injection of india ink in the ventral pancreatic duct delimits the region of the pancreas in which ventral-type islets are restricted. This region is vascularized by branches of superior mesenteric artery. *Left:* × 160; *Right:* × 2.0. (From Orci, ref. 33, with permission).

In the human pancreas, the sampling is necessarily based on procedures different from those used in laboratory animals; to search for two different islet types in the human pancreas, we have defined, in the autopsy room, a sampling protocol in which the entire pancreas is first cleaned from surrounding tissue and then divided in eight different regions (I to VIII), partly on anatomical grounds (Fig. 4, *top*) (6). Each of the eight regions is then assayed with the four antisera on successive serial sections to determine the pattern of islet immunofluorescence. In this way, we can reveal the presence of glucagon-rich islets in all eight regions of the pancreas; however, in regions I to IV of the pancreatic head, glucagon-rich islets were restricted to the anterior part of the horizontal slices. By contrast, pancreatic polypeptide-rich islets were observed exclusively in the posterior part of regions I to IV. These parts often constitute a lobe that can be cleaved from the pancreatic head (see Fig. 4) (7).

The heterogeneity of islets in the rodent and human pancreas is assumed to be linked to the dual origin of the gland during embryogenesis (8): the glucagon-rich islets would derive from the larger dorsal anlage, the pancreatic polypeptide-rich islets from the smaller ventral bud (Fig. 5). This hypothesis was recently supported in the human by the observation of a fetal annular pancreas. In this condition, characterized by the absence of rotation of the ventral bud that encircles the duodenum, four-fifths of the pancreatic tissue surrounding the duodenum ventrally shows pancreatic polypeptide immunofluorescence, whereas only the remaining one-fifth, situated dorsally, contains detectable glucagon (Fig. 6) (9). In the perspective of the known interactions between secretory cells of the islet (10–12) (see the section, Islet Cell Communication), one of the numerous questions that is raised is whether pancreatic polypeptide-rich islets respond differently than glucagon-rich islets to a glucose stimulus and/or whether there are specific stimuli for each islet type. The segregation of the two islet types in different regions of the pancreas renders possible their separate isolation for *in vitro* studies, and the assessment of morphological parameters linked to function in B cells from either glucagon-rich or pancreatic-polypeptide-rich islets during stimulation appears now feasible (13).

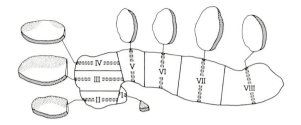

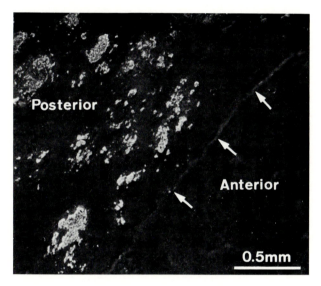

FIG. 4. Upper panel: Schematic representation of a human pancreas divided into the eight sampling regions (I to VIII). Regions I to IV constitute the pancreatic head, and each horizontal slice taken in these regions can be further subdivided into an anterior and posterior region (*stippled area*) on the basis of the distribution of pancreatic polypeptide cells. (From Malaisse-Lagae et al., ref 7, with permission). **Lower panel:** Example of an horizontal section through regions II, III, or IV following immunofluorescent staining of pancreatic polypeptide. Immunofluorescence is restricted to the posterior part of the section and is separated from the anterior, unstained part by a plane of connective tissue (*arrows*). The cleaving of the pancreatic head along this plane may yield a distinct lobe at the posterior aspect of the head containing most of the pancreatic polypeptide. × 36. (From Orci and Perrelet, ref. 4, with permission).

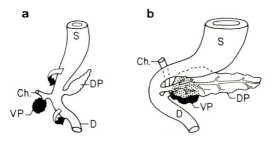

FIG. 5. Schematic drawing of the early **(a)** and late **(b)** positions of the ventral pancreatic bud (*in black*) during development. The ventral bud rotates behind the dorsal primordium to form the posterior lobe rich in pancreatic polypeptide (*black and stippled areas*). **(a)** = 5 mm embryo; **(b)** = 15 mm embryo. S = stomach; Ch = ductus choledocus; D = duodenum; VP = ventral pancreas; DP = dorsal pancreas. Note that in the rodent pancreas, the terminology "dorsal-" and "ventral-type islet" refers to the respective origin of the two islet types. (From Orci, ref. 33, with permission).

ISLET CELL COMMUNICATION

Besides the possible role of endocrine cell distribution in the regulation of islet secretion, the other pattern of islet structure that must be considered in this perspective is represented by specific plasma membrane domains, the nexus or gap junctions, between endocrine cells (Fig. 7). Such domains render direct cellular interactions possible through the exchange of certain molecules from one cytoplasm to the other; this process of intercytoplasmic exchange of ions or small molecules is called "intercellular coupling" and a review of its features will be found in the article by Hertzberg et al. (14). In the islet of Langerhans, gap junctions were identified not only between B cells, but also between A and B and/or B and D cells, in both

FIG. 6. Upper panel: Horizontal section through the duodenum **(D)** of a human fetus (11 cm) with an annular pancreas. The duodenum wall is entirely surrounded by pancreatic tissue and the *black rectangle* delimits a zone of merging (*dotted line*) between the pancreatic polypeptide-rich and the glucagon-rich regions. HE stain. × 18. **Middle and lower panels:** Zone of merging between the glucagon-rich and pancreatic polypeptide-rich regions following immunofluorescent staining with pancreatic polypeptide antiserum and glucagon antiserum, respectively; this shows the clearcut segregation of the two types of immunofluorescent cells. × 90. (From Stefan et al., ref. 9, with permission).

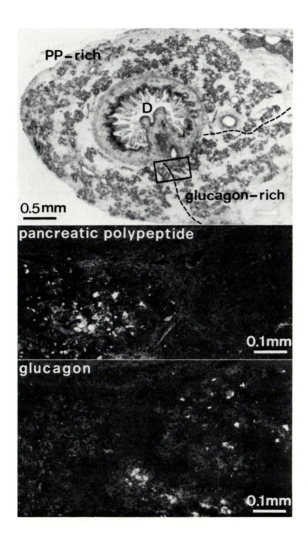

20   CELLULAR RELATIONSHIPS

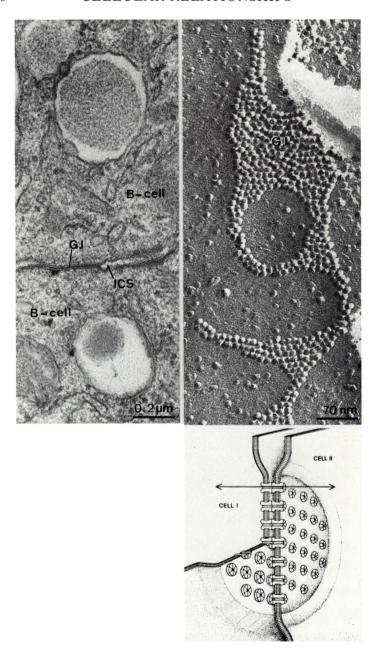

thin-section and freeze-fracture electron microscopy (15–18). The characterization of the coupling role of gap junctions requires electrophysiology and dye injection techniques. Electrophysiology enables one to detect the passage of ions between cells through the low-resistance pathway represented by gap junctions, a process named "electrical coupling," whereas dye injection allows the following of the exchange of small molecules through gap junctions, a process called "metabolic coupling." In microdissected mouse islets, electrical coupling was found to occur over several B-cell diameters (19,20), whereas in monolayer cultures of endocrine pancreas, the intracellular injection of a low-molecular weight fluorescent dye impermeant to the cell membrane showed a rapid spread of the staining to several adjacent cells without leaking in the extracellular space (21). The demonstration of an exchange of endogeneous molecules between pancreatic endocrine cells, the prerequisite for a possible regulatory role of gap junctions, succeeded in monolayer cultures of rat neonatal pancreas in which ^{3}H-uridine nucleotides were shown to migrate from cytoplasmically ^{3}H-uridine-labeled islet cells (donors) to neighboring, nuclearly ^{3}H-thymidine-labeled cells (recipients) (22,24). In both dye- and metabolite-transfer studies carried out in monolayer culture, not all islet cells present in a given cluster appeared coupled to each other at a given time. In a sample cluster, some cells did not exchange molecules with their neighbors, whereas other cells did, usually with two to eight adjacent cells. As a result of this limited exchange, small unconnected territories of coupled cells appeared in a cluster when several of its constituting cells were successively microinjected (Fig. 8). This finding suggests

←

FIG. 7. Right: Field from the peripheral cytoplasm of two B-cells in thin section electron microscopy. At the site labeled **GJ**, the two plasma membranes delimiting the cells come into very close proximity, almost obliterating the extracellular space (**ICS**). The region of close proximity between the two membranes represents a nexus or gap junction. × 61000. **Left:** Field of a B-cell plasma membrane in a freeze-fracture replica at a region of gap junction (**GJ**). The latter is represented by the close packing of intramembrane (protein) particles. Each particle is assumed to have an hexagonal configuration and to be in register with a similar particle in the neighboring membrane so as to delimit intercytoplasmic channels through which ions or small molecules can be exchanged (*arrow*). (Drawing modified from L.A. Staehelin and B.E. Hull (1978): Junction between living cells. *Sci. Am.*, 238:141–152.)

that a monolayer endocrine cell cluster is not homogeneous, but consists rather of an assembly of independent microcolonies, at least as far as gap junctional coupling is concerned. Whether or not similar territories of coupled cells exist in the intact islet remains to be established. In view of the heterogeneous population of endocrine cells forming the islets and of the possible functional interactions between these cells, a question of obvious importance was to determine whether or not gap junctions observed morphologically between heterologous cell

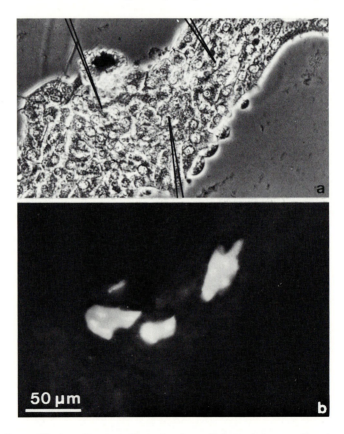

FIG. 8. a: Cluster of pancreatic endocrine cells in monolayer culture in which three injections (identified by the drawn *micropipettes*) of a fluorescent impermeant dye (carboxyfluorescein) have been carried out. **b:** Same cluster as shown above but visualized in fluorescent light. Each injection site has determined a fluorescent territory composed of several coupled cells but the three territories do not communicate with each other. × 330. (From Orci, ref. 33, with permission).

types were also mediating an heterologous metabolic coupling. Immunocytochemical demonstration and electron microscopical identification of communicating islet cells, following dye- or metabolite-transfer experiments, revealed that exogenous fluorescent dyes (in cells in culture and within isolated islets) and endogenous uridine nucleotides (in cultured cells) were exchanged not only between B cells, but also between A and B or D cells (25, 33). Besides the morphological demonstration of gap junctions between all cells of the islet of Langerhans and the identification of intercellular coupling with both exogenous and endogenous molecules, further evidence in support of a possible regulatory role of the coupling was the finding that gap junctions are modulated according to cell function. When the development of these junctions was assessed quantitatively (as the total area of the junctions and their number of constituting particles), in resting and in stimulated B cells, they could be shown to represent a very small fraction of the total B cell surface (0.02% to 0.04%, i.e., less than 0.2 μm^2) at rest, whereas stimulation of insulin secretion by glibenclamide increased both their size and frequency (28,29). Further, the size of gap junctions appeared inversely correlated with the insulin content of B cells (Fig. 9) (30). The assessment of functional coupling by electrophysiological and dye-injection techniques, during stim-

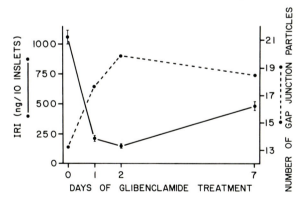

FIG. 9. Quantitation of gap junctional particles as seen in freeze-fracture replicas (cf. Fig. 7) on B-cell plasma membrane during depletion of insulin content by glibenclamide. Note the opposite increase of gap junction particles (a direct measure of gap junctional size and an indirect one of coupling) and decrease of insulin content over time. (From Meda et. al., ref. 30, with permission).

ulated insulin release, showed likewise evidence for increased communication in this condition (21). Clearly, the data on gap junctions and intercellular coupling among endocrine cells of the islet of Langerhans are abundant, but at the present time an integrative functional scheme for these data is lacking. What is now needed is the unambiguous evidence that intercellular coupling does participate in the normal functioning of the islet, and experiments to compare the secretory behavior of endocrine islet cells without junctions (i.e., isolated cells) and with junctions (on reaggregation of isolated cells) are an attempt in this direction (31).

CONCLUSION

We have shown that the islet of Langerhans and its *in vitro* model, the monolayer culture, possesses, in addition to a probable hormonal control via specific binding of active ligand(s) at the cell surface (32), at least two additional features that could participate in the modulation of the secretory response of its four constituting endocrine cells. These features are: (a) a precise topographical relationship of the different endocrine cell types one respective to the other, together with different proportions of glucagon- and pancreatic polypeptide cells depending on the anatomical location of the islet in the pancreas; and (b) the presence, between all islet cell types, of specific membrane differentiations, the nexus or gap junctions, which mediate the transfer of ions and small exogeneous and endogeneous molecules between adjacent endocrine cells. The understanding of all these possible regulatory influences will, it is hoped, evolve in a satisfactory model accounting for the adaptative secretory responses of the islet to a variety of metabolic situations.

ACKNOWLEDGMENTS

Most of the data presented in this chapter has been adapted from the Banting Memorial Lecture, 1981 (33).

This work was supported by the Swiss National Science Foundation, grant nr. 3.668.80 and 3.460.83, and by a subsidy from Hoechst Pharmaceuticals Ltd.

REFERENCES

1. Coons, A.H., Leduc, E.H., and Connolly, J. (1955): Studies on antibody production. I. A method for the histochemical demonstration of specific antibody and its application to a study of the hyperimmune rabbit. *J. Exp. Med.*, 102:49–63.
2. Orci, L., Baetens, D., Ravazzola, M., Stefan, Y., and Malaisse-Lagae, F. (1976): Pancreatic polypeptide and glucagon: non-random distribution in pancreatic islets. *Life Sci.*, 19:1811–1815.
3. Baetens, D., Malaisse-Lagae, F., Perrelet, A., and Orci, L. (1979): Endocrine pancreas: three dimensional reconstruction shows two types of islets of Langerhans. *Science*, 206:1323–1325.
4. Orci, L., and Perrelet, A. (1979): La microarchitecture des îlots de Langerhans. *Pour Sci.*, 22:30–44.
5. Orci, L., and Perrelet, A. (1981): The morphology of the A-cell. In: *Glucagon. Physiology, Pathophysiology and Morphology of the Pancreatic A-cells. Part I: Morphology*, edited by R.H. Unger and L. Orci, p. 1. Elsevier/ North Holland Biomedical Press, New York.
6. Orci, L., Malaisse-Lagae, F., Baetens, D., and Perrelet, A. (1978): Pancreatic-polypeptide-rich regions in human pancreas. *Lancet*, 2:1200–1201.
7. Malaisse-Lagae, F., Stefan, Y., Cox, J., Perrelet, A., and Orci, L. (1979): Identification of a lobe in the adult human pancreas rich in pancreatic polypeptide. *Diabetologia*, 17:361–365.
8. O'Rahilly, R., and Müller, F. (1978): A model of the pancreas to illustrate its development. *Acta Anat. (Basel)*, 100:380–385.
9. Stefan, Y., Grasso, S., Perrelet, A., and Orci, L. (1982): The pancreatic polypeptide-rich lobe of the human pancreas: definitive identification of its derivation from the ventral pancreatic primordium. *Diabetologia*, 23:141–142.
10. Orci, L., and Unger, R.H. (1975): Functional subdivision of islets of Langerhans and possible role of D-cells. *Lancet*, 2:1243–1244.
11. Unger, R.H., Dobbs, R.E., and Orci, L. (1978): Insulin, glucagon and somatostatin secretion in the regulation of metabolism. *Ann. Rev. Physiol.*, 40:307–343.
12. Unger, R.H., and Orci, L. (1981): Glucagon and the A cell. Physiology and pathophysiology (first of two parts). *N. Engl. J. Med.*, 304:1518–1524.
13. Trimble, E.R., and Renold, A.E. (1981): Ventral and dorsal areas of rat pancreas: islet hormone content and secretion. *Am. J. Physiol.*, 240:E422–E427.
14. Hertzberg, E.L., Lawrence, T.S., and Gilula, N.B. (1981): Gap junctional communication. *Ann. Rev. Physiol.*, 43:479–491.
15. Orci, L., Unger, R.H., and Renold, A.E. (1973): Structural coupling between pancreatic islet cells. *Experientia*, 29:1015–1018.
16. Orci, L., Malaisse-Lagae, F., Amherdt, M., Ravazzola, M., Weisswang, A., Dobbs, R., Perrelet, A., and Unger, R. (1975): Cell contacts in human islets of Langerhans. *J. Clin. Endocrinol. Metab.*, 41:841–844.

17. Orci, L., Malaisse-Lagae, F., Ravazzola, M., Rouiller, D., Renold, A.E., Perrelet, A., and Unger, R.H. (1975): A morphological basis for intercellular communication between A- and B-cells in the endocrine pancreas. *J. Clin. Invest.*, 56:1066–1070.
18. Orci, L., and Perrelet, A. (1977): Morphology of membrane systems in pancreatic islets. In: *The Diabetic Pancreas*, edited by B.W. Volk and K.F. Wellman, p. 171. Plenum Press, New York.
19. Meissner, H.P. (1976): Electrophysiological evidence for coupling between β-cells of pancreatic islets. *Nature*, 262:502–504.
20. Eddlestone, G.T., and Rojas, E. (1980): Evidence of electrical coupling between mouse pancreatic β-cells. *J. Physiol. (Lond.)*, 303:76P–77P.
21. Kohen, E., Kohen, C., Thorell, B., Mintz, D.H., and Rabinovitch, A. (1979): Intercellular communication in pancreatic islet monolayer cultures: a microfluorometric study. *Science*, 204:862–865.
22. Meda, P., Amherdt, M., Perrelet, A., and Orci, L. (1981): Metabolic coupling between cultured pancreatic B-cells. *Exp. Cell Res.*, 133:421–430.
23. Meda, P., Amherdt, M., Perrelet, A., and Orci, L. (1980): Coupling between insulin-containing cells. A morphological approach. In: *Diabetes 1979*, edited by W.K. Waldhäusl, Excerpta Medica ICS 500, p. 496. Elsevier/ North Holland, Amsterdam.
24. Meda, P., Perrelet, A., and Orci, L. (1982): Endocrine cell interactions in the islets of Langerhans. In: *Functional Integration of Cells in Animal Tissues*, edited by J.D. Pitts and M.E. Finbow, p. 113–131. Cambridge University Press, Cambridge.
25. Michaels, R.L., and Sheridan, J.D. (1981): Dye coupling among immunocytochemically distinct cell types. *Science*, 214:801–803.
26. Meda, P., Kohen, E., Kohen, C., and Orci, L. (1981): Couplage hétérocellulaire dans les cultures de cellules endocrines pancréatiques. *C.R. Acad. Sci. (Paris)*, 293:607–610.
27. Meda, P., Kohen, E., Kohen, C., Rabinovitch, A., and Orci, L. (1982): Direct communication of homologous and heterologous endocrine islet cells in culture. *J. Cell Biol.*, 92:221–226.
28. Meda, P., Perrelet, A., and Orci, L. (1979): Increase of gap junctions between pancreatic B-cells during stimulation of insulin secretion. *J. Cell Biol.*, 82:441–448.
29. Meda, P., Perrelet, A., and Orci, L. (1980): Gap junctions and B-cell function. *Horm. Metab. Res. (Suppl.)*, 10:157–162.
30. Meda, P., Halban, P., Perrelet, A., Renold, A.E., and Orci, L. (1980): Gap junction development is correlated with insulin content in pancreatic B-cell. *Science*, 209:1026–1028.
31. Halban, P.A., Wollheim, d.B., Blondel, B., Meda, P., Niesor, E.N., and Mintz, D.H. (1982): The possible importance of contact between pancreatic islet cells for the control of insulin release. *Endocrinology*, 111:86–94.
32. Patel, Y., Amherdt, M., and Orci, L. (1982): Quantitative electron microscopic autoradiography of insulin, glucagon and somatostatin binding sites on islets. *Science*, 217:1155–1156.
33. Orci, L. (1982): Macro- and micro-domains in the endocrine pancreas. Banting Lecture, 1981. *Diabetes*, 31:538–565.

… *The Importance of Islets of Langerhans for Modern Endocrinology*, edited by K. Federlin and J. Scholtholt, Raven Press, New York © 1984.

Evidence of a Glucose-Sensitive Process in the Beta Cell that Regulates Preferential Secretion of Newly Synthesized Insulin

Gerold M. Grodsky, Gerald Gold, Herbert D. Landahl, Mikhail L. Gishizky, and Robert E. Nowlain

Metabolic Research Unit and Department of Biochemistry and Biophysics, University of California, San Francisco, California 94143

Preferential secretion of newly synthesized insulin from pancreatic slices (14) or islets (3,5–7,10,23–25,31) has been previously observed in the Metabolic Research Unit at the University of California, San Francisco and other laboratories using pulse-labeling techniques. In these experiments, radioactive insulin was secreted at a higher fractional rate than immunoreactive insulin, and secreted insulin also had a higher specific activity than the average cellular insulin. Previous experiments suggested, moreover, that the degree of preferential secretion may be regulated (5,6,25). We have accumulated evidence that preferential secretion in the beta cell is both regulated by glucose and is the result of a novel cellular process, which we called "marking." Marking of newly labeled hormone for preferential release occurs after proinsulin biosynthesis, during a time that labeled hormone is primarily associated with the Golgi and forming secretory vesicles of the beta cell. Although a cellular process comparable to marking has not yet been described for other cells, there is evidence of regulation of preferential secretion with other compounds; placental lactogen (29), prolactin (30), parathyroid hormone (17), salivary amylase (26), pancreatic amylase (27), gonadotropin (13), vasopressin (22), thyroglobulin (21), and acetylcholine (2) also have been reported to be secreted nonrandomly in response to a variety of stimuli. Thus, the glucose-stimulated marking process in beta cells may have a parallel in several of the numerous types of secretory cells that are capable of diverting for immediate release newly synthesized products in response to their physiologic regulators.

METHODS

Detailed methods for the isolation, incubation, and labeling of islets, and the separation and purification of insulin and proinsulin separately from both the secreted and islet fractions have been reported (7) and will be described only briefly. Islets were isolated from fed, 300- to 350-g male Long-Evans rats by collagenase digestion (16) and used immediately. Batches of 100 to 250 islets each were incubated for 45 min at 37°C in buffer containing 20 mM glucose, and a 15-min labeling period in 20 mM glucose plus 400 µCi/ml ^{3}H-leucine followed. Buffers after the labeling period contained a variety of glucose concentrations and test compounds, but they always contained 0.2 mM leucine to prevent continued synthesis of radioactive proteins. Secreted insulin was collected in a series of windows after the islets were washed extensively with buffer; secreted samples, therefore, were noncumulative; the time of collection of secreted samples is specified in each experiment.

Insulin and proinsulin were purified without carrier after each secreted or islet sample was extracted overnight in acid-ethanol (4). Both hormone and precursor in the extract were precipitated at pH 5.3 by the addition of ethanol and ether, redissolved in buffer, and applied to anti-insulin columns, which were synthesized by coupling a crude globulin fraction from guinea pig antiporcine insulin serum to Sepharose 4B by a cyanogen bromide procedure (1). Bound insulin and proinsulin were eluted with 1 N acetic acid, concentrated, then separated from each other on a 1 × 110 cm column of Biogel P30. Specific activity of insulin was calculated as the radioactivity eluting in the insulin peak divided by the immunoreactive insulin applied to the column of Biogel P30. Therefore, there is a small (less than 10%) but constant error due to proinsulin in the applied sample.

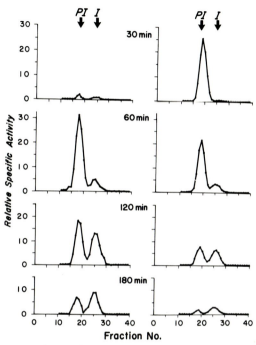

FIG. 1. Representative elution profiles from a Biogel P30 column. Islets were incubated continuously in 20 mM glucose beginning at −45 min, exposed to ^{3}H-leucine between 0 and 15 min, then incubated in buffer containing 0.2 mM leucine. Proinsulin and insulin in the islets or in noncumulative, secreted samples were extracted with acid-ethanol at the times specified. Hormones in the extracts were further purified without carrier by anti-insulin-Sepharose chromatography and Biogel P30 chromatography.

RESULTS AND DISCUSSION

Figure 1 is an example of a series of elution profiles obtained from columns of Biogel P30. Islets were continuously incubated in 20 mM glucose to establish steady-state conditions, and, for reference, labeling was done between min 0 and 15. Several of the processing, storage, and secretory characteristics of proinsulin and insulin are illustrated in this figure. First, at every time point there were only two peaks corresponding to proinsulin and insulin. Thus, as reported (28), preproinsulin is too transient to detect in this type of experiment. Secondly, there was an approximately 30-min period after labeling during which all radioactivity remained in proinsulin. Secretion of label during this period also was marginal. This 30-min period probably represents the transit time of labeled protein from the rough endoplasmic reticulum to the Golgi and forming secretory vesicles where conversion of proinsulin to insulin begins (15,28); a 30-min transit time also was reported in radioautographic studies for grains of leucine-labeled protein to appear over profiles of secretory granules (20). Thirdly, both insulin and proinsulin were secreted; the proportion of labeled pro- to mature hormone in the secreted fraction was similar to that within the islets at the same time. Thus, as reported (7,23), secretion was relatively independent of the storage form of the hormone in the secretory granule. Fourthly, by 60 min the specific activity of secreted insulin exceeded that of the average islet insulin. This is one indication of preferential release of newly synthesized insulin, which will be discussed in detail later. Finally, there was a time-dependent loss of almost all of the labeled hormones from the islets during the 3-h period of incubation.

Part of this loss was due to the conversion of proinsulin to insulin, in addition to secretion. Radioactivity contained in the excised C-peptide is eliminated during purification on anti-insulin columns. This loss can be corrected mathematically, as has been done for the scattergram in Fig. 2, which plots the kinetics of conversion of proinsulin to insulin. Conversion began approximately 30 min after the cessation of the pulse, indicating entry of labeled proinsulin into forming secretory granules. Once started, conversion progressed with a $t_{1/2}$ of approximately 50 min, as reported (28).

Whether or not a significant proportion of proinsulin is destroyed during conversion to insulin had not been previously addressed. Figure 3 shows the total amount of labeled proinsulin and insulin recovered from the islet plus secreted fractions. Although most of the labeled proinsulin disappeared

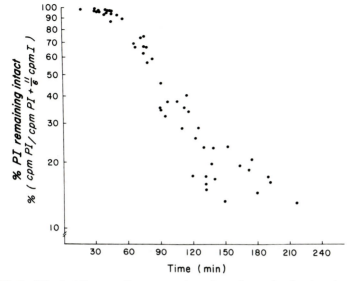

FIG. 2. Effect of time on the conversion of newly synthesized proinsulin to insulin. Islets were incubated continuously in 20 mM glucose beginning at −45 min and exposed to ^{3}H-leucine between 0 and 15 min. Samples were obtained by extracting the islets and accumulated incubation buffer together. The radioactivity eluting from columns of Biogel P30 in the insulin peak was multiplied by 11/6 to correct for the difference in leucine content between insulin and proinsulin. (From Gold et al., ref. 7, with permission).

during these incubations, the lost label was almost totally recovered in insulin, as indicated by a near-constant sum of radioactivity found in the two proteins. Thus, during glucose stimulation, labeled proinsulin is almost stoichiometrically converted to insulin. Degradation of either or both hormones was too slow to measure accurately in these experiments, in accordance with a reported insulin degradation rate in glucose-stimulated islets of less than 0.6%/h (11).

The above figures provide a quantitative and kinetic overview of labeled hormone transport, processing, and storage in the beta cell. However, this overview does not apply to all immunoreactive hormone because, as previously mentioned, labeled hormone and prohormone were secreted at a higher fractional rate than the average, immunoreactive insulin (data not shown) (7), and the specific activity of secreted insulin exceeded that of the average cellular insulin by threefold (Fig. 4b). Note that as

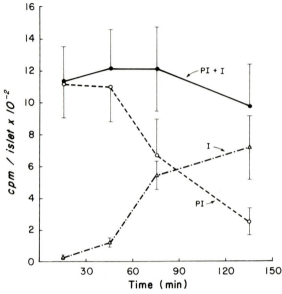

FIG. 3. Effect of time on the recovery of proinsulin and insulin in the islets plus incubation buffer. Samples were obtained from islets, which were incubated continuously in 20 mM glucose beginning at −45 min and exposed to ^{3}H-leucine between 0 and 15 min. The radioactivity eluting from columns of Biogel P30 in the insulin peak was multiplied by 11/6 to correct for the difference in leucine content between insulin and proinsulin. Points represent the mean + SE from six experiments. (From Gold et al., ref. 7, with permission).

soon as there was elevated secretion of labeled hormone, there also was evidence of preferential secretion. Figure 4a is a series of hypothetical specific activity versus time relationships predicted from a steady-state model describing heterogeneous insulin synthesis, storage, and transit through the beta cell (7). Labeled hormone was considered to enter three different sized compartments of preferentially released insulin in these equations. Note that the maximal size of the preferentially secreted compartment can be approximated visually because it is inversely related to the ratio of maximal specific activities of secreted versus cellular insulin. By mathematical or visual inspection, the observed datum from glucose-stimulated islets most closely resembled the curves for a compartment containing as much as 33% of the total islet insulin. In addition, islets

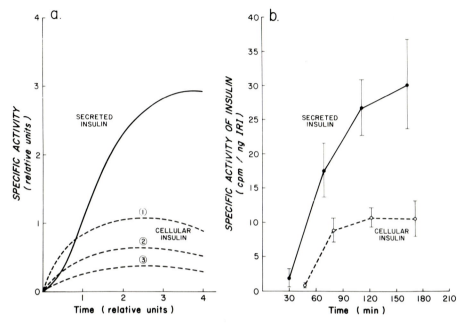

FIG. 4. Effect of time on the predicted and experimentally determined specific activity of secreted and cellular insulin. In **a**, steady-state equations were used to predict and relationships between the specific activity of secreted and cellular insulin if the percentage of total islet insulin contained in the glucose-labile compartment was 33% in No. 1, 20% in No. 2, and 11% in No. 3. In **b**, experimental data were obtained from islets continuously incubated in 20 mM glucose beginning at −45 min and exposed to ^{3}H-leucine between 0 and 15 min. Islets were washed twice with buffer before a 20-min sample of secreted hormone was collected. Points representing secreted hormone are drawn at the center of the 20-min interval, and all points represent the mean + SE from eight experiments. (From Gold et al., ref. 7, with permission).

separated from either the dorsal or ventral portion of the pancreas also secreted insulin with a specific activity threefold above that of the average cellular insulin. Therefore, both had comparably sized compartments, and preferential secretion was not simply the result of rapid synthesis and secretion of insulin in either of these functionally and compositionally distinct islets (data not shown) (7).

The same steady-state equations used to estimate compartment size were also used to predict the flow of radioactive hormone through the cellular organelles involved with protein synthesis, storage, and secretion. In Fig. 5, our predicted data were drawn on top of a bar graph of the histological distribution with time of radioactive grains in the beta cells of fetal rat pancreas incubated with ^{3}H-leucine (adapted from data published in ref. 20). Despite geographic and experimental differences, there is excellent agreement. As anticipated from experiments of the conversion of proinsulin to insulin and the onset of secretion of labeled hormone, after 40 min the rough endoplasmic reticulum was largely depleted and the secretory granules were filling with labeled hormone. Note that after the pulse, a considerable quantity of labeled hormone resides in the Golgi for more than 40 min.

We recently observed that the glucose concentration in the incubation buffer during the period of time that radioactive

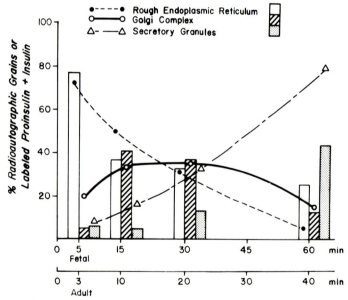

FIG. 5. Effect of time on the predicted and determined distribution of radioactive proinsulin and insulin in the RER, Golgi, and secretory vesicles of the beta cell, which is drawn on top of the actual distribution of radioactive grains over the organelles of fetal rat pancreas incubated with ^{3}H-leucine (20). Two time scales are drawn because the predicted distribution used equations describing synthesis, storage, and secretion of insulin in islets from mature rats, and the histologic distribution was determined for beta cells from fetal rat pancreas.

hormone was in the Golgi and forming secretory vesicles significantly affected the specific activity of hormone later released in response to a variety of stimuli (6). An example is shown in Fig. 6. After labeling, islets were incubated in either 2 or 20 mM glucose for this critical time (marking period), then returned to 20 mM glucose. If a low concentration of glucose was present during the marking period, near-random release followed, and secreted insulin had a specific activity comparable to that of the

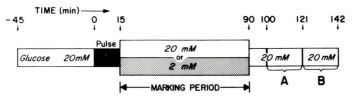

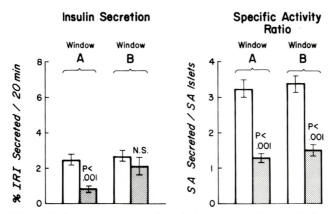

FIG. 6. Effect of glucose concentration during the marking period on the secretion rate and specific activity ratio between secreted and cellular insulin. Islets were incubated in 20 mM glucose beginning at −45 min and exposed to ^{3}H-leucine between 0 and 15 min. After labeling, islets were washed twice with buffer, then either marked by incubation in 20 mM glucose or not marked by incubation in 2 mM glucose from min 15 to 90. Both groups were washed twice with buffer at 90 min and identically incubated in 20 mM glucose for the duration of the experiment. Noncumulative samples of secreted insulin were collected after buffer was removed and islets were washed with buffer. All buffers after the labeling period contained 0.2 mM leucine. Insulin from secreted and islet samples was purified by acid-ethanol extraction, affinity chromatography and chromatography on columns of Biogel P30. Bars represent the mean + SE from nine experiments.

average cellular insulin. However, if islets were marked during this period by exposure to elevated glucose, preferential release followed, as indicated by a specific activity ratio (specific activity of secreted insulin/specific activity of the average cellular insulin) of more than three. This difference probably does not reflect altered provision of label into secretory vesicles because the glucose concentration did not affect the cellular conversion of labeled proinsulin to insulin (data not shown).

Also, once marking has or has not occurred, the degree of preferential secretion does not appear to depend significantly on the glucose concentration, secretion rate, or secretagogue after the marking period. Essentially, the same pattern of preferential or near-random secretion was observed when any of the following secretagogues was used after the marking period: 5 mM glucose; 5 mM glucose + 100 µg/ml tolbutamide; 2 mM glucose + 50 mM potassium; or 20 mM glucose + 1 mM 3-isobutyl-1-methylxanthine. Therefore, a glucose-sensitive event or events in the marking period were the primary determinants of the specific activity of insulin later to be mobilized for secretion.

The most important portion of the marking period was investigated further by exposing islets to elevated concentrations of glucose during either the early or the later part of this 75-min marking interval. An event or events that subsequently led to preferential secretion occurred primarily in the early part of the marking period; however, the glucose concentration during the later part of the marking period also affected the degree of preferential secretion (data not shown). The early part of the marking period corresponds closely with the time that radioactive protein is in the Golgi and forming secretory vesicles.

The secretory mechanism of the beta cell is not clearly defined, but microtubules have been implicated in this process (19), and an interaction between forming secretory granules and the microtubular network could provide the mechanism for preferential release. An experiment is shown in Fig. 7 in which assembled microtubules were disrupted with 0°C temperature after the marking period, followed by sufficient time at 37°C for reestablishment of microtubular structures (18). Dissolution

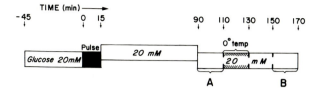

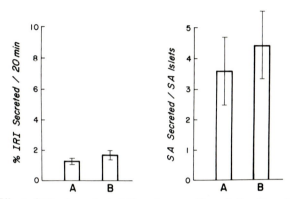

FIG. 7. Effect of 20-min period at 0° on the specific activity of insulin secreted from previously marked islets. Islets were incubated continuously in 20 mM glucose beginning at −45 min and exposed to ^{3}H-leucine between 0 and 15 min. After labeling, islets were marked by incubation at 37° in 20 mM glucose until 90 min, chilled to 0° from 110 to 130 min, then returned to incubation at 37° for the duration of the experiment. Noncumulative samples of secreted insulin were collected at the specified times after buffer was removed and islets were washed with buffer. All buffers after the labeling period contained 0.2 mM leucine. Insulin from secreted and islet samples was purified by acid-ethanol extraction, affinity chromatography and chromatography of columns of Biogel P30. Bars represent the mean + SE from four experiments.

and reformation of microtubules should randomize secretion from marked islets if specific sets of microtubules mediate the marking process; however, cold had no randomizing effect.

The cellular mechanism for selective mobilization and secretion of newly synthesized insulin from marked islets remains unknown. The critical marking period comprises the time of transit of proinsulin to the Golgi and the approximate time required to convert half of this proinsulin to insulin—both events associated with functions of the Golgi and forming secretory vesicles. The effect of glucose on the beta cell during this period may modify the functional efficacy or the sorting properties of the Golgi, resulting in a secretory vesicle that has enhanced secretory competency, or it may activate a novel, regulated secretory route. Despite uncertainty about how the beta cell accomplishes preferential secretion, glucose-stimulated marking may represent one of the cellular mechanisms for altering the overall secretory rate of immunoreactive insulin in response to conditions that produce time-dependent (8,9) or chronic modulation (12).

SUMMARY

1. After a 30-min period associated with cellular transport from the rough endoplasmic reticulum to the Golgi, proinsulin is almost stoichiometrically converted to insulin in a pseudo-first-order process with a $t_{1/2}$ of approximately 50 min.

2. Both newly synthesized proinsulin and insulin are secreted without preference to the storage form of the hormone in the secretory vesicle.

3. Labeled hormone is secreted preferentially from glucose-stimulated islets obtained from either the entire pancreas or only the dorsal or ventral region.

4. The preferentially secreted compartment could contain as much as 33% of the total islet insulin (estimated from a steady-state mathematical model).

5. Preferential secretion reflects a cellular marking process, which is sensitive to the glucose concentration of the incubation medium after the period of labeling and before the period of secretion.

6. Kinetic experiments also suggest that marking occurs primarily when the radioactive protein is in the Golgi and in forming secretory vesicles.

7. Preferential secretion may not require specific sets of intact microtubules because disruption of microtubules by a 20-min period at 0°C did not affect preferential secretion from previously marked islets.

ACKNOWLEDGMENTS

This work was supported in part by National Institutes of Health grants AM01410 and AM21933. Mikhail L. Gishizky is a recipient of an Achievement Rewards for College Scientists (ARCS) Fellowship, Northern California Chapter.

REFERENCES

1. Berne, C. (1975): Anti-insulin serum coupled to Sepharose 4B as a tool for the investigation of insulin biosynthesis in the B-cells of obese hyperglycemic mice. *Endocrinology*, 97:1241–1247.
2. Collier, B. (1969): The preferential release of newly synthesized transmitter by a sympathetic ganglion. *J. Physiol. (Lond.)*, 205:341–352.
3. Creutzfeldt, C., Track, N. S., and Creutzfeldt, W. (1973): In vitro studies of the rate of proinsulin and insulin turnover in seven human insulinomas. *Eur. J. Clin. Invest.*, 3:371–384.
4. Davoren, P. R. (1962): The isolation of insulin from a single cat pancreas. *Biochim. Biophys. Acta*, 63:150–153.
5. Gold, G., Reaven, G. M., and Reaven, E. P. (1981): Effect of age on proinsulin and insulin secretory patterns in isolated rat islets. *Diabetes*, 30:77–82.
6. Gold, G., Gishizky, M. L., and Grodsky, G. M. (1983): Evidence that glucose "marks" beta cells resulting in preferential release of newly synthesized insulin. *Science*, 218:56–58.
7. Gold, G., Landahl, H. D., Gishizky, M. L. and Grodsky, G. M. (1982): Heterogeneity and compartmental properties of insulin storage and secretion in rat islets. *J. Clin. Invest.*, 69:554–563.
8. Grill, V., Adamson, U., and Cerasi, E. (1978): Immediate and time-dependent effects of glucose on insulin release from rat pancreatic tissue— evidence for different mechanisms of action. *J. Clin. Invest.*, 61:1034–1043.
9. Grodsky, G. M., Landahl, H. D., Curry, D., and Bennett, L. (1970): In vitro studies suggesting a two-compartmental model of insulin secretion. In: *The Structure and Metabolism of the Pancreatic Islets*, edited by S. Falkmer, B. Hellman, and I. B. Taljedal, pp. 409–421. Pergamon Press, Oxford.
10. Gutman, R. A., Fink, G., Shapiro, J. R., Selawry, H., and Recant, L. (1973): Proinsulin and insulin release with a human insulinoma and adjacent nonadenomatous pancreas. *J. Clin. Endocrinol. Metab.*, 36:978–987.
11. Halban, P. A., and Wollheim, C. B. (1980): Intracellular degradation of insulin stores by rat pancreatic islets in vitro: an alternative pathway for homeostasis of pancreatic insulin content. *J. Biol. Chem.*, 255:6003–6006.
12. Hedeskov, C. (1980): Mechanism of glucose induced insulin secretion. *Physiol. Revs.*, 60:442–509.
13. Hoff, J. D., Lasley, B. L., Wang, C. F., and Yen, S. S. C. (1977): Two pools of pituitary gonadotropin: regulation during the menstrual cycle. *J. Clin. Endocrinol. Metab.*, 44:302–312.
14. Howell, S. L., Parry. D. G., and Taylor, K. W. (1965): Secretion of newly synthesized insulin in vitro. *Nature (Lond.)*, 208:487.
15. Kemmler, W., Steiner, D. F., and Borg, J. (1973): Studies on the

conversion of proinsulin to insulin. III. Studies in vitro with a crude secretion granule fraction isolated from rat islets of Langerhans. *J. Biol. Chem.*, 248:4544–4551.
16. Lacy, P. E., and Kostianovsky, M. (1967): Method for the isolation of intact islets of Langerhans from the rat pancreas. *Diabetes*, 16:35–39.
17. MacGregor, R. R., Hamilton, J. W., and Cohn, D. V. (1975): The by-pass of tissue hormone stores during the secretion of newly synthesized parathyroid hormone. *Endocrinology*, 97:178–188.
18. McLean, W. G., and Keen, P. (1973): Colchicine-binding activity and neurotubule integrity in a rat sympathetic ganglion. *Exp. Cell Res.*, 80: 345–353.
19. Malaisse-Lagae, F., Amherdt, M., Ravazzola, M., Sener, A., Hutton, J. C., Orci, L. and Malaisse, W. J. (1979): Role of microtubules in the synthesis, conversion and release of (pro)insulin. *J. Clin. Invest.*, 63: 1284–1296.
20. Orci, L., Lambert, A. E., Kanazawa, Y., Amherdt, M., Rouiller, C., and Renold, A. E. (1971): Morphological and biochemical studies of B cells of fetal rat endocrine pancreas in organ culture: evidence for (pro) insulin biosynthesis. *J. Cell Biol.*, 50:565–582.
21. Rosenberg, L. L., LaRoche, G., and Ehlert, J. M. (1966): Evidence for heterogeneous turnover of iodine in rat thyroid glands. *Endocrinology*, 79: 927–934.
22. Sachs, J., Fawcett, P., Takabatake, Y., and Portanova, R. (1969): Biosynthesis and release of vasopressin and neurophysin. *Recent Prog. Horm. Res.*, 25:447–491.
23. Sando, H., Borg, J., and Steiner, D. F. (1972): Studies on the secretion of newly synthesized proinsulin and insulin from isolated rat islets of Langerhans. *J. Clin. Invest.*, 51:1476–1485.
24. Sando, H., and Grodsky, G. M. (1973): Dynamic synthesis and release of insulin and proinsulin from perifused islets. *Diabetes*, 22:354–360.
25. Schatz, H., Nierle, C., and Pfeiffer, E. F. (1975): (Pro-) insulin (biosynthesis and release of newly synthesized (pro-) insulin) from isolated islets of rat pancreas in the presence of amino acids and sulphonylureas. *Eur. J. Clin. Invest.*, 5:477–485.
26. Sharoni, Y., Eimerl, S., and Schramm, M. (1976): Secretion of old versus new exportable protein in rat parotid slices: control by neurotransmitters. *J. Cell Biol.*, 71:107–122.
27. Slaby, F., and Bryan, J. (1976): High uptake of myo-inositol by rat pancreatic tissue in vitro stimulates secretion. *J. Biol. Chem.*, 251: 5078–5086.
28. Steiner, D. F., Kemmler, W., Clark, J. L., Oyer, P. E., and Rubenstein, A. H. (1972): The biosynthesis of insulin. In: *Handbook of Physiology, Endocrinology, Sect. 7 Vol. 1*, edited by D. F. Steiner, and N. Freinkel, pp. 175–198. Williams and Wilkins, Baltimore, Md.
29. Suwa, S., and Friesen, H. (1969): Biosynthesis of human placental proteins and human placental lactogen (HPL) in vitro. II. Dynamic studies of normal term placentas. *Endocrinology*, 85:1037–1045.
30. Swearingen, K. C. (1971): Heterogeneous turnover of adenohypophysial prolactin. *Endocrinology*, 89:1380–1388.
31. Track, N. S. (1977): Insulin biosynthesis. In: *Insulin and Metabolism*, edited by J. S. Bajaj, pp. 13–39. Excerpta Medica, Amsterdam.

The Importance of Islets of Langerhans for Modern Endocrinology, edited by K. Federlin and J. Scholtholt, Raven Press, New York © 1984.

Subunit Structures and Actions of the Receptors for Insulin and the Insulin-like Growth Factors

Michael P. Czech, Joan Massague, Kin Yu, Catherine L. Oppenheimer, and Cristina Mottola

Department of Biochemistry, University of Massachusetts Medical Center, Worcester, Massachusetts 01605

The receptor systems that mediate the biological actions of insulin and the insulin-like growth factors I and II (IGF I and IGF II) comprise a useful model system for studies on transmembrane signaling as well as receptor–receptor interactions. It has been known for some time that these three hormones contain a high degree of sequence homology in their structures (24,25). Interestingly, these homologies have been found to extend to both structural and functional aspects of these hormones' receptors and signaling systems in target cells. We have used these receptor systems for the study of structure-function relationships in hormone signaling, and we will summarize in this chapter several of the general concepts that have developed from these studies.

Figure 1 summarizes some of the general physiological features of the membrane effector systems and biological effects of these hormones. The effects of insulin on major target tissues, such as muscle and adipose tissue, involve at least two cellular domains—the intracellular cytoplasm and the plasma membrane. Many of the effects of insulin on cellular transporters and enzymes are rapid and fully reversible on removing hormone. They are fully expressed within minutes after addition of hormone. Whereas the mechanism of action of insulin on membrane components, such as the hexose transporter, is not fully understood, the hormone actions on intracellular enzymes appear to reflect changes in phosphorylation state of these proteins (4). Paradoxically, some enzymes are dephosphorylated in response to insulin action (e.g., glycogen synthase and pyruvate dehydrogenase), whereas other cellular proteins appear to be phosphorylated in response to insulin action (the S-6 ribosomal protein and ATP-citrate lyase). Any detailed mechanism of insulin action will have to account for this apparently paradoxical phenomenology.

There are at least two levels at which these actions of insulin interface with the actions of the insulin-like growth factors. First, as indicated in Fig. 1, the receptors for these ligands show cross-reactivity in binding kinetics (23). Thus, insulin has been shown to inhibit the binding of the labeled insulin-like growth factors to cell receptors when the former unlabeled ligand is added at high concentrations. Similarly, high concentrations of either IGF I or IGF II have been shown to inhibit insulin-receptor interaction. Therefore, the concept has developed that the receptors for insulin and the IGFs exhibit high affinity for a specific ligand and lower but distinct affinities for the other ligands as well.

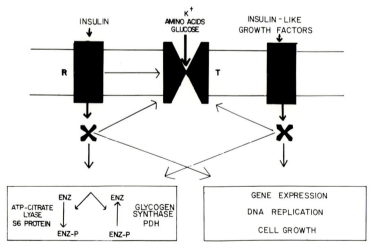

FIG. 1. General relationships between the membrane signaling systems for insulin and the insulin-like growth factors.

A second level of interaction among these systems is at the level of biological responsiveness. The classical response to the IGFs involves stimulation of cell proliferation or thymidine incorporation into DNA; however, it has been recently appreciated that at least in some cell types this response can also be observed with insulin (19). The concentrations of insulin required to generate these effects vary among cell types, indicating that in certain cases the insulin receptor may mediate such effects, and in other cases the insulin-like growth factor receptors may mediate insulin action on cell proliferation. Conversely, several instances in which the IGFs stimulate the rapid effects associated with insulin action have been discovered. Again, many of these effects have been thought to be mediated by the insulin receptor because of the high concentrations of IGFs required (13).

Given the above general considerations and issues, our own studies have focused on three principle questions related to insulin and insulin-like growth factor actions:

1. What are the receptor structures that are involved in binding the three partially homologous peptide hormones?

2. What specific biological responses are linked to each of the receptor structures identified?

3. Are the actions of these receptor systems coordinated or linked by mechanisms that allow one receptor to modulate the activity of another?

IDENTIFICATION OF RECEPTOR STRUCTURES

Methodologies developed over the last several years have allowed the insulin receptor to be isolated or identified by a variety of techniques. Affinity purification using immobilized insulin preparations was developed over a decade ago by Cuatrecasas and colleagues (2) and is still employed for insulin receptor purification. The low abundance of this receptor in target tissues has allowed only relatively small amounts of receptor to be purified by this methodology. However, Jacobs and colleagues (9,10) and Siegel et al. (27) isolated microgram amounts of receptor by this method and have succeeded in characterizing the subunit structure of purified receptor. An alternative method that has become very useful involves the use of anti-receptor antibodies obtained from patients with acanthosis nigricans and insulin resistance (7). These antibodies have been shown to be directed against the insulin binding site on the receptor and thus will block insulin binding. Immunoprecipitation of the insulin receptor from detergent extracts has been successful using these antibodies, and characterization of the insulin receptor subunits has been possible (7). In addition, it has been possible to take advantage of the characteristic receptor structure in order to purify insulin receptor by the two-dimensional gel electrophoresis (8). This method has also proved valuable in identifying insulin receptor subunits and performing peptide mapping of the subunits. As yet, there has been no successful purification of the receptors for the IGFs.

Affinity labeling technology has succeeded in identification of insulin receptor and IGF receptor subunits. Experiments in our laboratory demonstrated the utility of two different strategies for affinity labeling these receptors by employment of chemical cross-linkers. Using disuccinimidyl suberate or its analogs, we were able to selectively cross-link ^{125}I-insulin to its specific receptor in a variety of tissues. This cross-linker also effectively affinity labeled the receptors for IGF I and IGF II in later studies (11,12,16,20). Success in affinity labeling the insulin receptor and the IGF I receptor was also demonstrated using photoactive analogs of the peptide hormones (1,28). Thus, over the past few years, a large number of techniques have been applied to the problem of identifying and characterizing these receptor systems.

Experiments using both affinity purification techniques and affinity cross-linking have independently led to a hypothetical model of the insulin receptor subunit structure that is consistent with virtually all of the available literature. These results have been reviewed in detail previously (6,10). Briefly, a key finding was that the insulin receptor complex existed as a high molecular weight disulfide-linked component in target cell membranes (9,22). Addition of reducing agents dissociated a receptor complex migrating in the 350,000 dalton range on dodecyl sulfate gels into receptor subunits of 125,000 and 90,000 daltons. A lower molecular weight species that resulted from a reduction of the native disulfide-linked complex appears to result from intrinsic proteolytic cleavage of the receptor structure in cell membranes (17). We denote the identified insulin receptor subunits as α and β, respectively (18). A key finding was that incubation of insulin receptor in low concentrations of reductant dissociated the receptor into a partially reduced fragment, which migrated on gels with an apparent molecular weight of 210,000. When this partially reduced fragment was run on a second dimension gel in the presence of high concentrations of reductant, it dissociated into both α and β subunit species. Since this partially reduced receptor fragment was about half the molecular weight of the total receptor complex, it was hypothesized that the native complex consisted of two partially reduced fragments. This hypothesis was strongly supported by two-dimensional analysis of the receptor forms that had been generated by proteolytic nicking of the β subunit (17,18). Thus, the proposed receptor structure is illustrated in Fig. 2 and represents a heterotetrameric disulfide-linked complex containing a total of four subunits—two α and two β subunit species. Other data gathered indicated that both subunits contained oligosaccharide (10). Interestingly, this structure for the native receptor complex reinforces the possibility that the receptor structure is divalent, i.e., it binds to more than one insulin molecule.

A striking aspect of further experimentation in this area was the finding that a receptor with high affinity for IGF I exhibited structural characteristics very similar to the insulin receptor. Both the native receptor for IGF I and the resident α and β subunits that were disulfide linked within the structure migrated on dodecyl sulfate gels at the same apparent molecular weights as was found for the insulin receptor. Furthermore, all of the characteristic responses of the receptor structure to incubation with reductant or other experimental manipulations parallel those found for the insulin receptor (20). When the α and β subunits as isolated on dodecyl sulfate gels from both insulin and IGF I receptors are incubated with thrombin, the resulting fragmentation maps are identical for the respective subunits in each receptor. These data raise the possibility that the insulin and IGF I receptor proteins are the products of a common gene and that post-translational modification changes their affinities for insulin and IGF I. Further structural data will be required to clarify this issue. At this point, it can be said with reasonable confidence that these two receptor structures as shown in Fig. 2 are strikingly similar and cannot be differentiated at the level of resolution provided by dodecyl sulfate gel electrophoresis.

A receptor structure with highest affinity for IGF II was also

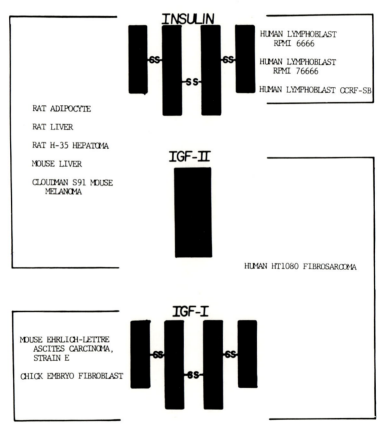

FIG. 2. Proposed minimum subunit structures of the receptors for insulin, IGF I and IGF II. The receptors for insulin and IGF I are composed of 125,000 dalton (α) and 90,000 dalton (β) disulfide-linked subunits, whereas the IGF II receptor protein that has been identified is about 250,000 daltons.

identified by affinity cross-linking technology (11,16,20). This receptor structure has no detectable disulfide-linked subunits and exhibits a molecular weight on dodecyl sulfate gels that varies between approximately 230,000 and 270,000. This receptor is not a proteolytic fragment of the IGF I receptor because several tissues can be observed to contain this receptor in the absence of the IGF I receptor structure. Using the affinity labeling procedures, the relative affinities of each of the three receptor structures for insulin and the IGFs could be determined by employing unlabeled ligand to compete for labeling of the receptor for ^{125}I-hormone. These studies indicated that the insulin receptor species exhibited the highest affinity for insulin and much lower affinity for the IGFs. The IGF I receptor exhibited the highest affinity for IGF I, lower affinity for IGF II, and the lowest affinity for insulin. The IGF II receptor structure exhibited high affinity for IGF II, lower affinity for IGF I, and no detectable affinity for insulin. It should be noted that some heterogeneity of binding kinetics could be observed for these structures among the different tissues studied, although the relative affinities for the three ligands remains essentially constant. The available data would indicate that the three receptor structures for insulin and the IGFs that are represented in Fig. 2 can account for all of the biological effects known that are elicited by these three peptide hormones (5).

THE BIOLOGICAL ACTIONS OF INSULIN AND THE IGF RECEPTOR STRUCTURES

Although significant progress had been made in defining which biological responses were linked to the insulin versus IGF receptors prior to identifying the receptor structures (23), the availability of affinity labeling techniques for the receptors has significantly enhanced our information on this issue. The strategy that we have used in our own studies has been to study the biological actions of these receptors in cell types that contain only one or two of the three possible receptor structures. In this way, each receptor structure can be studied independently from the influence of the other receptor structures on a given biological response. In screening a large number of primary tissues and cell lines in culture, we found a large number that contained all three receptor structures in varying amounts. These included human fibroblast, the rat L-6 myoblast cell line, rat and human lymphocyte cell lines, rat and human placenta, and several human melanoma cell lines. Of greater interest were those cell lines depicted in Fig. 2 that contain the one or two receptor structures that are within the brackets. Two of the classical target tissues for insulin—adipocytes and liver—contain the insulin and IGF II receptor structures but not the IGF I receptor.

Because the IGFs activate the rapid hexose transport and enzymatic responses in adipocytes only at concentrations above those which saturate their own receptors, it could be concluded that the IGF II receptor structure does not modulate these acute responses classically associated with insulin action. Because liver and fat cells could not be used to assess the effectiveness of the IGF I receptor to mediate actions on these acute responses, isolated soleus muscles were employed. We had more difficulty performing these studies since skeletal muscles contain all three receptor structures. However, by carefully assessing the dose-response relationships between ligand concentration and hexose and amino-acid transport activation, we could again demonstrate the impotence of the IGF II receptor to activate these responses (29). In contrast, the IGF I receptor structure that is homologous to the insulin receptor structure was found to be linked to these rapid biological responses in muscle (29). Consequently, the two receptor structures that are structurally similar appear to mediate similar biological responses in relation to acute effects.

This similarity appears not to be the case in relation to the effects on DNA replication and cellular proliferation. We could demonstrate in strain E of the Ehrlich-Lettre ascites carcinoma cell line that contain only the IGF I receptor (with extremely little or no insulin receptor) that the IGF I receptor was fully competent to mediate the growth effects (*unpublished*). Other studies have indicated that this receptor species is also capable of mediating growth in human fibroblasts, but in this cell type the insulin receptor is impotent in mediating growth effects. In contrast, we were able to demonstrate that the insulin receptor was quite potent in mediating growth effects in H-35 hepatoma cells (19). Thus, we conclude that the IGF I receptor seems linked to cell proliferation, whereas the insulin receptor varies in this capability depending on the cell type in which it resides. The IGF II receptor appears to be capable of mediating effects of DNA replication but the results available to date are not unequivocal. Table 1 summarizes the capabilities of these three receptors to modulate biological responses.

TABLE 1. *Biological responses of the receptors for insulin and the insulin-like growth factors*

Hormone	Apparent receptor mass (K)	Acute effects in adipocytes or muscle	Effects on DNA replication
Insulin	350–400	Yes	Some cell lines
IGF I	350–400	Yes	Yes
IGF II	250	No	Probably, but not unequivocally documented

RECEPTOR–RECEPTOR INTERACTIONS

The similarities noted above on both structural and functional aspects of the receptor systems for insulin and the IGFs suggest that there might be a high degree of coordination among these receptor systems. In concert with this notion, an effect of insulin to increase the binding of ^{125}I-IGF II to isolated fat cells was reported (26). The advent of affinity labeling methodology for the identification of the IGF II receptor and the finding that adipocytes contain only insulin and IGF II receptors allowed more recent definitive analysis of this phenomenon (19,21). The effect of insulin on the IGF II receptor was shown to be rapid, temperature dependent, and consistent with a physiological dose-response relationship for insulin (14,21). Interestingly, it could be shown that the effect of insulin only could be observed in intact cells (adipocytes or H-35 hepatoma cells) but was not observed when the hormone was added directly to isolated membranes (19). Furthermore, the increased IGF II binding to its receptor reflected solely an increase in affinity of its receptor with no apparent change in the receptor number upon Scatchard analysis (21).

The characteristic response of the IGF II receptor to insulin action is extremely similar to that observed for hexose transport activation. Both of these membrane components that exhibit sensitivity to insulin action are modulated within minutes at 37°, exhibit in the range of 10-fold effects by insulin, and appear to be fully reversible on washing cells free of insulin. However, recent evidence has suggested that the hexose transport activity is activated by insulin by a mechanism that involves increasing the number of transporters in the cell surface membrane. Therefore, Cushman and colleagues discovered that [^{3}H] cytochalasin B binding, an estimate for the number of D-glucose transporters, was increased in the plasma membrane fraction of cells that had been treated with insulin (3). Concomittantly, a decrease in the number of transporters was observed in a light microsomal fraction that these investigators suggested may be an intracellular membrane fraction. Independent studies by Kono's laboratory have also paralleled these basic observations using reconstitution methodology (15).

The above results would seem to indicate a difference between the mechanism of activation of the IGF II receptor, which appears to be purely an affinity change, and the hexose transport system, which appears to be involved in a membrane recycling phenomenon. Recent studies in our own laboratory have indicated that the dynamics of activation of these two systems may be much more complicated than the above concepts. When we compared the state of the IGF II receptor in isolated membrane fractions from cells treated in the presence or absence of insulin, we discovered that the homogenization process itself converts the IGF II receptor in control cells to the high affinity state (21). Thus, no change in affinity is observed because of insulin action in intact cells when binding measurements are made in the isolated membrane fractions.

Perhaps more interesting was our observation that the apparent number of IGF II receptors was markedly increased in the plasma membrane fraction of insulin-treated cells, whereas a significant decrease in receptor number was observed in the low-density microsome fraction. Therefore, whereas in the intact cell, insulin action on the IGF II receptor was visualized as solely an affinity change, in isolated membranes the effect of insulin was visualized solely as a redistribution of receptor numbers, as is the case for the hexose transporter. These phenomena have yet to be clarified in terms of mechanism. One possibility to explain these results is that homogenization of cells may fragment or shear certain critical cell surface microdomains that form low-density vesicles and migrate with the Golgi fraction on sucrose density gradients. If insulin were to stabilize such microdomains in addition to its direct activation of these sensitive membrane components, then the apparent redistribution that is observed could be explained. Further experiments will have to be performed to determine the underlying mechanisms involved in these systems.

CONCLUSIONS

Affinity labeling and affinity cross-linking techniques have successfully identified three receptor structures that bind with high affinity to insulin, IGF I, or IGF II and that can account for the known biological effects of these peptide hormones. The receptor structures for insulin and IGF I appear maximally to be heterotetrameric disulfide-linked complexes containing two subunit types and are extremely similar to each other in structure. The responsiveness of tissues and cell lines to insulin and the IGFs depend on the specific receptor structures present on the cell surface as well as the biological effectiveness of each of these receptor structures on specific biological pathways. The receptors for insulin and IGF I appear to be capable of activating the rapid transport and enzyme modulations that are classically associated with insulin action, whereas the receptor for IGF II is impotent in mediating these effects. The IGF I receptor, and probably the IGF II receptor, mediate DNA replication and cell proliferation, whereas the insulin receptor is capable of mediating these types of effects in certain cell types only. The regulatory actions of the three receptors identified may be highly coordinated in that insulin action rapidly increases the affinity of the IGF II receptor for IGF II by an unknown mechanism. This effect of insulin may allow direct actions on transport and enzyme functions via its own receptor and indirect actions to promote growth effects through the IGF II receptor.

REFERENCES

1. Bhaumick, B., Bala, R., and Hollenberg, M. (1981): Somatomedin receptor of human placenta: solubilization, photolabeling, partial purification, and comparison with insulin receptor. *Proc. Natl. Acad. Sci. USA*, 78:4279–4283.
2. Cuatrecasas, P., and Hollenberg, M. (1976): Membrane receptors and hormone action. In: *Advances in Protein Chemistry 30*, edited by C. F. Anfinsen, J. T. Edsall, and F. M. Richards, pp. 251–451. Academic Press, New York.
3. Cushman, S., and Wardzala, L. (1980): Potential mechanism of insulin action on glucose transport in the isolated rat adipose cell. *J. Biol. Chem.*, 255:4758–4762.
4. Czech, M. (1977): Molecular basis of insulin action. *Ann. Rev. Biochem.*, 46:359–384.
5. Czech, M. (1982): Structural and functional homologies in the receptors for insulin and the insulin-like growth factors. *Cell*, 31:8–10.
6. Czech, M., Massague, J., and Pilch, P. (1981): The insulin receptor: structural features. *Trends in Biochem. Sci.*, 6:222–225.
7. Harrison, L., and Itin, A. (1980): Purification of the insulin receptor from human placenta by chromatography on immobilized wheat germ lectin and receptor antibody. *J. Biol. Chem.*, 255:12066–12072.
8. Heinrich, J., and Czech, M. (1982): Insulin receptor structure and purification. In: *Receptors for Polypeptide Hormones*, edited by Barry I. Posner. Marcel Dekker, New York (*in press*).
9. Jacobs, S., Hazum, E., and Cuatrecases, P. (1980): The subunit structure of rat liver insulin receptor. *J. Biol. Chem.*, 255:6937–6940.
10. Jacobs, S., and Cuatrecasas, P. (1981): Insulin receptor: structure and function. *Endocr. Rev.*, 2:251–263.
11. Kasuga, M., Van Obberghen, E., Nissley, P., and Rechler, M. (1981): Demonstration of two subtypes of insulin-like growth factor receptors by affinity crosslinking. *J. Biol. Chem.*, 256:5305–5308.
12. Kasuga, M., Van Obberghen, E., Nissley, P., and Rechler, M. (1982): Structure of the insulin-like growth factor receptor in chicken embryo fibroblasts. *Proc. Natl. Acad. Sci. USA*, 79:1864–1868.
13. King, G., Kahn, R., Rechler, M. and Nissley, P. (1980): Direct demonstration of separate receptors for growth and metabolic activities of insulin and multiplication-stimulating activity using antibodies to the insulin receptor. *J. Clin. Invest.*, 66:130–140.
14. King, G., Rechler, M., and Kahn, R. (1982): Interactions between the receptors for insulin and the insulin-like growth factors on adipocytes. *J. Biol. Chem.*, 257:10001–10006.
15. Kono, T., Robinson, F., Blevins, T., and Ezaki, O. (1982): Evidence

that translocation of the glucose transport activity is the major mechanism of insulin action on glucose transport in fat cells. *J. Biol. Chem.*, 257:10942–10947.
16. Massague, J., Guillette, B., and Czech, M. (1981): Affinity labeling of multiplication stimulating activity receptors in membranes from rat and human tissues. *J. Biol. Chem.*, 256:2122–2125.
17. Massague, J., Pilch, P., and Czech, M. (1981): A unique proteolytic cleavage site on the β subunit of the insulin receptor. *J. Biol. Chem.*, 256:3182–3190.
18. Massague, J., Pilch, P., and Czech, M. (1981): Electrophoretic resolution of three major insulin receptor structures with unique subunit stoichiometries. *Proc. Natl. Acad. Sci. USA*, 77:7127–7141.
19. Massague, J., Blinderman, L. and Czech, M. (1982): The high affinity insulin receptor mediates growth stimulation in rat hepatoma cells. *J. Biol. Chem.*, 257:13958–13963.
20. Massague, J., and Czech, M. (1982): The subunit structures of two distinct receptors for insulin-like growth factors I and II and their relationships to the insulin receptor. *J. Bio. Chem.*, 257:5038–5045.
21. Oppenheimer, C., Pessin, J., Massague, J. Gitomer, W., and Czech, M. (1983): Insulin action rapidly modulates the apparent affinity of the insulin-like growth factor II receptor. *J. Biol. Chem.*, 258:4824–4830.
22. Pilch, P., and Czech, M. (1980): The subunit structure of the high affinity insulin receptor. *J. Biol. Chem.*, 255:1722–1731.
23. Rechler, M., Nissley, P., King, G., Moses, Al., Van Obberghen-Schilling, E., Romanus, J., Knight, A., Short, P. and White, R. (1981): Multiplication stimulating activity from the BRL 3A rat liver cell line: relation to human somatomedins and insulin. *J. Supramol. Struct.*, 15:253–286.
24. Rinderknecht, E., and Humbel, R. (1978): Primary structure of human insulin-like growth factor II. *FEBS Letts.*, 89:283–286.
25. Rinderknecht, E., and Humbel, R. (1978): The amino acid sequence of human insulin-like growth factor I and its structural homology with proinsulin. *J. Biol. Chem.*, 253:2769–2776.
26. Schloenle, E., Zapf, J., and Froesch, E. (1977): Effects of insulin and NSILA on adipocytes of normal and diabetic rats: receptor binding, glucose transport, and glucose metabolism. *Diabetologia*, 13:243–249.
27. Siegel, T., Ganguly, S., Jacobs, S., Rosen, O., and Rubin, C. (1981): Purification and properties of the human placental insulin receptor. *J. Biol. Chem.*, 256:9266–9273.
28. Yip, C., Moule, M., and Yeung, C. (1982): Subunit structure of insulin receptor of rat adipocytes as demonstrated by photoaffinity labeling. *Biochemistry*, 21:2940–2945.
29. Yu, K., and Czech, M. (1982): The type I insulin-like growth factor mediates the stimulatory effects of multiplication stimulating activity on hexose and amino acid transport in rat soleus muscle. *J. Biol. Chem.*, (*submitted*).

The Importance of Islets of Langerhans for Modern Endocrinology, edited by K. Federlin and J. Scholtholt, Raven Press, New York © 1984.

Gastrointestinal Hormones and Islet Function

Werner Creutzfeldt

Department of Medicine, University of Göttingen, 3400 - Göttingen, Federal Republic of Germany

A review of the effect of gastrointestinal hormones on islet function is appropriate in this volume because Ernst Pfeiffer and his group have contributed so much to this field since 1964. Some of these contributions are discussed in detail in this chapter.

INCRETIN

The term "incretin" has been used for many years for a humoral factor contained in the intestinal tract that releases insulin or potentiates the glucose-induced insulin release. The first who suggested this was Moore in 1906, who also speculated, long before the isolation of insulin, that diabetes may be due to the absence of an intestinal excitant (22). La Barre, the great Belgian physiologist, did his cross-circulation experiments with crude extracts containing secretin (18). He was able to demonstrate a blood glucose lowering effect of these extracts and concluded that they contained one stimulant for the exocrine pancreas and another for the endocrine pancreas and called this latter fraction "incretin."

The whole story was forgotten for 20 years but became again of interest to the scientific world when in 1964, McIntyre, Holthworth, and Turner (21) and, at the same time, Elrick and co-workers (13) demonstrated that an intraduodenal glucose load, which even does not increase blood glucose as much as a small i.v. glucose load, releases much more insulin than this i.v.

glucose load. This potential of an oral stimulus has been called since that time the "incretin effect." A few years later, Roger Unger named the connection between the gut and the islets the "enteroinsular axis" (33). We have to realize that this axis is rather complex and comprises substrate stimulation from the nutrients directly to the islets with their different cells, neurotransmission, and endocrine transmission (4). The neurotransmission has been well demonstrated in the last several years by using transplanted pancreas or isolated transplanted islets, showing that in these denervated preparations, the insulin release after food intake is much reduced. In 1973, a paper on this topic from Ernst Pfeiffer's laboratory demonstrated that atropine diminished the insulin response to oral glucose and intraduodenal amino acids, and also significantly decreased the insulin-releasing potency of impure CCK (26).

SECRETIN

All known gastrointestinal hormones have been investigated for their insulin-releasing potency due to the interest in the enteroinsular axis, which began with McIntyre's and Elrick's work. One of the very first who was exploring this field with pure hormones or nearly pure hormones was Ernst Pfeiffer in the years 1964 and 1965 (24). Figure 1 shows his discovery that *in vitro* secretin releases insulin. It is a perfect demonstration of an effect of a gastrointestinal hormone on insulin release. The judgement of this finding has changed over time. It is evident in Fig. 1 that rather arbitrary dosages of secretin were used. These are certainly by far exceeding the physiological plasma levels of secretin. If one uses such amounts of secretin, one can easily demonstrate an insulin release in man and even a blood glucose lowering effect (11). But this is pharmacology and not physiology. Furthermore, Boden has demonstrated in dogs after establishment of a sensitive and specific radioimmunoassay for secretin that one cannot release secretin by glucose (1). This is necessary for a substance to be fully recognized as an incretin because the effect of McIntyre and Elrick was demonstrated with glucose. The question whether or not the dose of secretin necessary to release insulin is in the physiological range has been

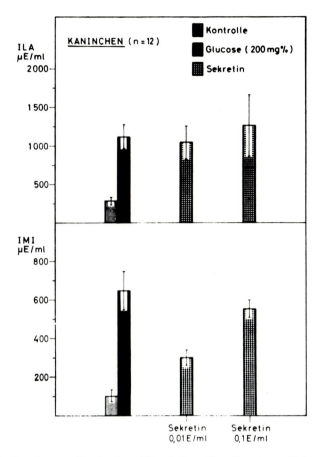

FIG. 1. Insulin secretion *in vitro*: Stimulation of insulin release (ILA = insulin-like activity; IMI = immunomeasurable insulin) from slices of rabbit pancreas incubated in buffer, in buffer + 200 mg/dl d-glucose, in buffer + 0.01 U secretin/ml and in buffer + 0.1U secretin/ml. Glucose-independent stimulation of insulin secretion by secretin to the same extent as with glucose. (From Pfeiffer et al., ref. 24, with permission).

decided by the experiments of Fahrenkrug and the Copenhagen group (13). If during a permanent glucose infusion HCl is given intraduodenally, one sees an increase of insulin and at the same time an increase of secretin, which suggests that both events are connected. However, if exogenous secretin is given in an amount that reproduces an identical secretin peak, no insulin release occurs. That result means that the increase of insulin after intraduodenal HCl instillation must be related to something else. In this context, it is of interest that with intraduodenal infusion of high doses of HCl, one can release GIP in man and rat (11). In the rat, GIP released by HCl enhances the insulin secretion induced by i.v. infusion of glucose, i.e., it has an incretin effect (11).

GASTRIN-CCK FAMILY

Secretin is a potent insulin releaser, but not a physiological incretin, like the gastrin-CCK family. Gastrin also releases insulin. However, Rehfeld and Stadil (28) have demonstrated that a significant response of insulin only occurs with dosages of gastrin that are high up in the super-physiological range. In addition, gastrin is released only very little by glucose, much better of course by protein, and so it may be an incretin after protein intake. More recent work of the Copenhagen group suggests that tetragastrin (the C-terminal tetrapeptide of CCK) is present in nerve terminals of the islets and as a neurotransmitter involved in the secretion of insulin (27).

CCK has been used in the 1960s by many authors and also by Ernst Pfeiffer's group for demonstrating insulin release. CCK is a very potent insulin releaser, if one uses impure preparations, which were the usual CCK preparations until 1975. Brown and co-workers were the first to demonstrate that one can abolish the incretin effect of CCK by purification (2). Ten percent pure CCK, this was the usually CCK preparation available from the Karolinska Institute, has an excellent incretin effect. In experiments by Thomas and co-workers (32), it has been demonstrated that different amino acids have different effects on the exocrine pancreas and the GIP release. The authors applied one perfusate into the duodenum that had little effect on GIP and insulin but a very strong effect on exocrine pancreatic secretion. Another perfusate, composed by different amino acids, released very well GIP and insulin but had little effect on the exocrine pancreas. These results clearly connect endogenous GIP but not endogenous CCK to amino-acid-induced insulin release. The purest form of CCK, the octapeptide of CCK, has in high dosages an effect on insulin secretion and even a stronger effect on glucagon secretion, but this effect disappears if one approaches nearly physiological dosages (15). In the isolated perfused porcine pancreas, different concentrations of porcine CCK-octapeptide in the physiological range had no effect on insulin secretion with different concentrations of glucose present in the perfusate and also no effect on glucagon secretion (20).

GIP

John Brown originally isolated as a side fraction from porcine intestinal extracts a peptide of the glucagon-secretin family that he and Viktor Mutt called "gastric inhibitory polypeptide." Since Brown was interested in a substance that inhibited gastric secretion, he used as a biological marker for concentrating and isolating this factor the inhibition of secretion in the Heidenhain pouch of dogs. This gave the substance its name. But soon, especially after the experiments of John Dupré, it was realized that the more interesting effect of this peptide is the potentiation of glucose-induced insulin release. This has been demonstrated *in vivo* (7) and *in vitro* (30) and in the isolated perfused pancreas (23).

GIP is released by glucose, protein, fat, and also acid. The fact that GIP releases insulin only in the presence of elevated glucose levels is apparently of clinical significance in order to prevent hypoglycemia (4). Another important protection against hypoglycemia is the capacity of insulin to inhibit GIP release in a kind of feedback control (2,3,6). Many functions of the gastrointestinal tract are controlled by feedback systems, like acid and gastrin release. The feedback control of fat-induced GIP secretion by insulin is impaired in obesity and glucose intolerance and can be restored by food restriction (10). We have demonstrated also the inhibitory effect of insulin on GIP release in juvenile type diabetics who were off insulin for 24 hr (16). However, this has been recently debated (34).

By discussing this controversy, I have to mention one of the significant contributions Ernst Pfeiffer made to clinical diabetology, i.e., the artificial pancreas, the Biostator®. Using this device, Verdonk, Service, and Go denied the existence of this feedback control mechanism between GIP and insulin (34). With the help of the Biostator®, the authors clamped the blood glucose and infused saline or insulin. They found no difference in the GIP response to triglycerides with or without insulin.

By reading their experimental set-up, we have considered the possibility that hyperinsulinemic clamping of the blood glucose masks the responsiveness of the GIP cells to insulin. This hypothesis could be proven by using the Biostator® for hyperinsulinemic and normoinsulinemic clamping for 2 hrs. Thereafter, 100-g triglycerides were ingested by the volunteers and the hyperinsulinemic clamping continued, respectively started (Fig. 2). If insulin is elevated 2 hrs before the fat meal, one sees no difference between the GIP response without and with insulin. But if the insulin infusion is started in the moment the fat load is given, then the GIP response is significantly suppressed (31). This demonstrates two things: (a) insulin does inhibit fat-

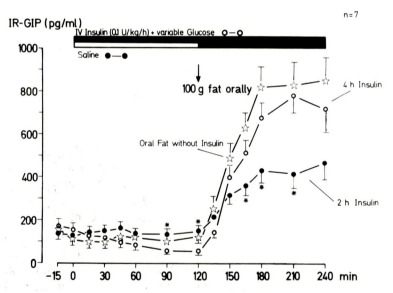

FIG. 2. IR-GIP response to ingestion of fat during saline infusion for 4 hr, insulin infusion for 4 hr (0.1 U/kg/hr) and during infusion of saline for 2 hr and insulin infusion during the next 2 hr. 100-g triglycerides were ingested 2 hr after start of the experiment. Blood glucose was clamped at the fasting level by glucose infusion using the Biostator®. (From Stöckmann et al., ref. 31, with permission).

induced GIP secretion in man, and (b) glucose clamping by simultaneous infusion of glucose and insulin may mask insulin effects if one loads the system too early with insulin. Whether this is due to the affinity of the receptors or negative cooperativity, I leave to the reader's judgement.

CHRONIC PANCREATITIS

There is another interesting contribution of Ernst Pfeiffer's group to the understanding of the enteroinsular axis. In 1971, it was published that, in contrast to normal animals, rats with pancreatic duct ligation did not respond to secretin injection with an insulin release, whereas they responded well to glucose (16) (Fig. 3). The authors speculated about a dependence of the endocrine on the exocrine pancreas, which was not functioning anymore if the exocrine pancreas was destroyed, and have reported about similar findings in patients with chronic pancreatitis. But these data have been debated (17). In the same

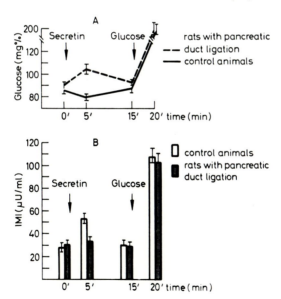

FIG. 3. Effect of i.v. injection of secretin and glucose on blood glucose and insulin release in rats with ligated pancreatic ducts (n = 18) and in control animals (n = 19) (means ± SEM). (From Creutzfeldt et al., ref. 5, with permission).

context, Pfeiffer's group explored the question whether or not an incretin effect still exists in chronic pancreatitis (25). They showed that a very special group of patients with chronic pancreatitis and normal i.v. glucose tolerance have much less insulin release after oral glucose than controls (Fig. 4). This raises the question whether or not in chronic pancreatitis a gut factor is lacking or the B cells are nonresponsive to incretin. We have tried to answer this question but did not have the same sort of patients under our care. However, while studying GIP and insulin release in chronic pancreatitis patients with steator-

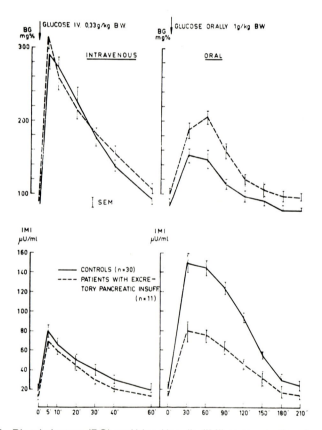

FIG. 4. Blood glucose (BG) and blood insulin (IMI) concentrations in patients with excretory pancreatic insufficiency (n = 11) and in normal controls (n = 30) (mean ± SEM) following i.v. and oral glucose loads. (From Raptis et al., ref. 25, with permission).

rhea but without overt diabetes, we could demonstrate that in this group the release of GIP in response to a test meal is impaired (8). Addition of pancreatin to the test meal significantly enhances the GIP release and the insulin response (Fig. 5). Simultaneously also, the glucose tolerance is much improved by just giving pancreatin. That means that GIP is only released after absorption of the food, and for this pancreatin is necessary in case of exocrine pancreatic insufficiency. This is a special

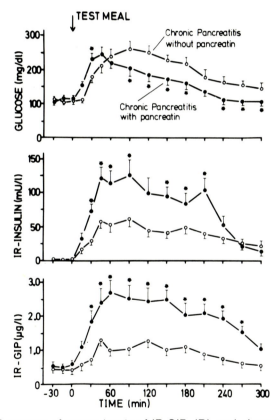

FIG. 5. Response of serum levels of IR-GIP, IRI, and glucose to a liquid mixed test meal given at time zero in 16 patients with chronic pancreatitis and massive steatorrhea. The test was performed once without and on a second occasion with pancreatin (9.0 g) given 5 min before ingestion of the test meal. Asterisks indicate significant difference between the two tests ($p < 0.05$ or less). ●—● with pancreatin, ○—○ without pancreatin. (From Ebert and Creutzfeldt, ref. 8, with permission.)

form of diabetes that corresponds to Moore's hypothesis (22) that in some diabetics a duodenal factor may lack which is responsible for their diabetes.

RECENT FINDINGS

So far, I have discussed the possible role of secretin, gastrin, CCK, and GIP as possible incretins, i.e., physiological releasers of insulin after food ingestion. I have not mentioned VIP (vasoactive intestinal peptide) because this peptide that belongs also to the secretin family is *not* a hormone but a neurotransmitter. It is only found in nerves and not in epithelial cells (19). I also have not discussed somatostatin, which is found in epithelial cells in the islets and the gut. I believe that this inhibitory peptide has mainly or even exclusively paracrine, i.e., local effects on the islets, and is not part of the enteroinsular axis.

However, I would like to point out that the strong case I have made for GIP may not be the final word in the incretin story. This statement is based on several recent findings. First, we have not been able to completely abolish the incretin effect of HCl or glucose in rats by infusing GIP antibodies (11,9). Second, others could not imitate the incretin effect of oral glucose by infusing glucose together with GIP in an amount that raised GIP plasma levels to the same extent as an oral glucose load (29). Third, we have recently studied the effect of i.v. infusion of gut extracts on the insulin-releasing effect of i.v. glucose. These gut extracts increased significantly the insulin release of glucose and at the same time lead to an increase of plasma GIP. After eliminating GIP from these extracts by immunoabsorption, no

FIG. 6. Effect on plasma levels of glucose, IRI, and IR-GIP in rats of an i.v. glucose load (1 g/kg/hr) (○—○), i.v. glucose plus gut extract (●—●), or i.v. glucose plus GIP-free gut extract (△—△). GIP was removed from the intestinal extracts by means of immunoabsorption. Both, the GIP-containing and the GIP-free extracts were adjusted to give an infusion rate of 37 mg protein/kg/hr. Each curve represents the mean ± SEM of twelve experiments. *Asterisk* indicates significant differences ($p < 0.05$ or less) between GIP-free and GIP-containing extracts. *Plus sign* indicates significant differences ($p < 0.02$ or less) between the control animals receiving glucose alone and the group receiving GIP-free gut extracts. (From Ebert et al., ref. 12, with permission).

increase of plasma GIP occurs after infusion of the extract, whereas a significant incretin effect is still present (Fig. 6), proving that a GIP-free gut extract still has incretin activity (12). This finding can be explained in two ways: either all the known gut hormones together have an incretin effect that cannot be abolished by taking out GIP or the small intestine contains unknown substances which create similar incretin activity as GIP.

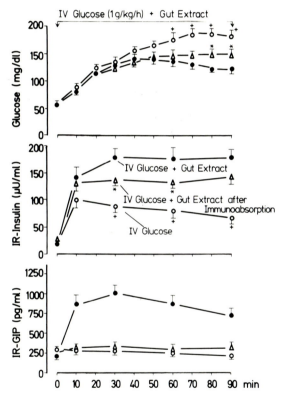

CONCLUSIONS

Our present knowledge about the relationship between gastrointestinal hormones and insulin secretion can be summarized as follows:

1. Secretin is not a physiological incretin.

2. The CCK family (CCK-4, -8, -33, -39 and gastrin) is without significance for insulin release induced by glucose ingestion. Its role as a neurotransmitter or as an interaction with other gastrointestinal hormones needs further investigation.
3. VIP is not a hormone and its role as a neurotransmitter has been unexplored.
4. GIP is a physiological incretin. Its release is regulated by nutrient absorption and negative feedback control via insulin.
5. There are still unknown incretins and there is a possibility of a combined action of several gastrointestinal hormones.
6. Somatostatin influences islet function via local (paracrine) secretion.

REFERENCES

1. Boden, G., Essa, N., Owen, O. E., and Reichle, F. A. (1974): Effects of intraduodenal administration of HCl and glucose on circulating immunoreactive secretin and insulin concentrations. *J. Clin. Invest.*, 53: 1185–1193.
2. Brown, J. C., Dryburgh, J. R., Ross, S. A., and Dupré, J. (1975): Identification and actions of gastric inhibitory polypeptide. *Recent Prog. Horm. Res.*, 31:487–532.
3. Cleator, J. G. M., and Gourlay, R. H. (1975): Release of immunoreactive gastric inhibitory polypeptide (IR-GIP) by oral ingestion of food substances. *Am. J. Surg.*, 130:128–135.
4. Creutzfeldt, W. (1979): The incretin concept today. *Diabetologia*, 16: 75–85.
5. Creutzfeldt, W., Talaulicar, M., Ebert, R., and Willms, B. (1980): Inhibition of gastric inhibitory polypeptide (GIP) release by insulin and glucose in juvenile diabetes. *Diabetes*, 29:140–145.
6. Crockett, S. E., Cataland, S., Falko, J. M., and Mazzaferri, E. L. (1976): The insulinotropic effect of endogenous gastric inhibitory polypeptide in normal subjects. *J. Clin. Endocrinol. Metab.*, 42:1098–1103.
7. Dupré, J., Ross, S. A., Watson, D., and Brown, J. C. (1973): Stimulation of insulin secretion by gastric inhibitory polypeptide in man. *J. Clin. Endocrinol. Metab.*, 37:826–828.
8. Ebert, R., and Creutzfeldt, W. (1980): Reversal of impaired GIP and insulin secretion in patients with pancreatogenic steatorrhea following enzyme substitution. *Diabetologia*, 19:198–204.
9. Ebert, R., and Creutzfeldt, W. (1982): Influence of GIP antiserum on glucose-induced insulin secretion in rats. *Endocrinology*, 111:1601–1606.
10. Ebert, R., Frerichs, H., and Creutzfeldt, W. (1979): Impaired feedback control of fat induced gastric inhibitory polypeptide (GIP) secretion by insulin in obesity and glucose intolerance. *Eur. J. Clin. Invest.*, 9:125–135.

11. Ebert, R., Illmer, K., and Creutzfeldt, W. (1979): Release of gastric inhibitory polypeptide (GIP) by intraduodenal acidification in rat and man and abolishment of the incretin effect of acid by GIP-antiserum in rats. *Gastroenterology*, 76:515–523.
12. Ebert, R., Unger, H., and Creutzfeldt, W. (1983): Preservation of incretin activity after removal of GIP from rat gut extracts by immunoabsorption. *Diabetologia*, 24:449–454.
13. Elrick, H., Stimmler, L., Hlad, C. J., and Arai, Y. (1964): Plasma insulin responses to oral and intravenous glucose administration. *J. Clin. Endocrinol. Metab.*, 24:1076–1082.
14. Fahrenkrug, J., Schaffalitzky de Muckadell, O. B., and Kühl, C. (1978): Effect of secretin on basal- and glucose stimulated insulin secretion in man. *Diabetologia*, 14:229–234.
15. Frame, C. M., Davidson, M. B., and Sturdevant, R. A. L. (1975): Effects of the octapeptide of cholecystokinin on insulin and glucagon secretion in the dog. *Endocrinology*, 97:549–553.
16. Goberna, R., Fussgänger, R. D., Raptis, S., Telib, M., and Pfeiffer, E. F. (1971): The role of the exocrine pancreas in the stimulation of insulin secretion by intestinal hormones. *Diabetologia*, 7:68–72.
17. Kalk, W. J., Vinik, A. I., Botha, J. L., Keller, P., and Jackson, W. P. U. (1975): Insulin responses to crude cholecystokinin-pancreozymin in normal subjects, in patients with chronic pancreatitis and patients with mild maturity onset diabetes. *J. Clin. Endocrinol. Metab.*, 41:172–176.
18. La Barre, J. (1936): *La sécretine: son rôle physiologique, ses propriétés thérapeutiques*. Masson, Paris.
19. Larsson, L. I. (1980): Gastrointestinal cells producing endocrine, neurocrine and paracrine messengers. *Clin. Gastroenterol.*, 9:485–516.
20. Lindkaer Jensen, S., Rehfeld, J. F., Holst, J. J., Vagn Nielsen, O., Fahrenkrug, J., and Schaffalitzky de Muckadell, O. B. (1981): Secretory effects of cholecystokinins on the isolated perfused porcine pancreas. *Acta Physiol. Scand.*, 111:225–232.
21. McIntyre, N., Holdworth, C. D., and Turner, D. S. (1964): New interpretation of oral glucose tolerance. *Lancet*, 2:20–21.
22. Moore, B., Edie, E. S., and Abram, J. H. (1906): On the treatment of diabetes mellitus by acid extract of duodenal mucous membrane. *Biochem. J.*, 1:28–38.
23. Pederson, R. A., and Brown, J. C. (1976): The insulinotropic action of gastric inhibitory polypeptide in the perfused isolated rat pancreas. *Endocrinology*, 99:780–785.
24. Pfeiffer, E. F., Telib, M., Ammon, J., Melani, F., and Ditschuneit, H. (1965): Direkte Stimulierung der Insulin-Sekretion in vitro durch Sekretin. *Dtsch. Med. Wochenschr.*, 38:1663–1669.
25. Raptis, S., Rau, R. M., Schröder, K. E., Hartmann, W., Faulhaber, J.-D., Clodi, P. H., and Pfeiffer, E. F. (1971): The role of exocrine pancreas in the stimulation of insulin secretion by intestinal hormones. *Diabetologia*, 7:160:167.
26. Raptis, S., Dollinger, H., Laube, H., Rau, R. M., Schröder, K. E., and Pfeiffer, E. F. (1973): Der Einfluß von Atropin auf die durch intestinale

Hormone induzierte Insulin sekretion des Menschen. *Res. Exp. Med. (Berl.)*, 160:234–247.
27. Rehfeld, J. F., Larsson, L. -I., Goltermann, N. R., Holst, J. J., Jensen, S. L., and Morley, J. S. Schwartz, T. W. (1980): Neural regulation of pancreatic hormone secretion by the C-terminal tetrapeptide of CCK. *Nature*, 284:33–38.
28. Rehfeld, J. F., and Stadil, F. (1973): The effect of gastrin on basal- and glucose-stimulated insulin secretion in man. *J. Clin. Invest.*, 52:1415–1426.
29. Sarson, D. L., Wood, S. M., Holder, D., and Bloom, S. R. (1982): The effect of glucose-dependent insulinotropic polypeptide infused at physiological concentrations on the release of insulin in man. *Diabetologia*, 22:33–36.
30. Schauder, P., Brown, J. C., Frerichs, H., and Creutzfeldt, W. (1975): Gastric inhibitory polypeptide: effect on glucose-induced insulin release from isolated rat pancreatic islets in vitro. *Diabetologia*, 11:483–484.
31. Stöckmann, F., Ebert, R., and Creutzfeldt, W. (1981): Hyperinsulinism during glucose clamping prevents demonstration of feedback regulation of GIP by insulin. *Diabetologia*, 21:331
32. Thomas, F. B., Sinar, D., Mazzaferri, E. L., Cataland, S., Mekhjian, H. S., Caldwell, J. H., and Fromkes, J. J. (1978): Selective release of gastric inhibitory polypeptide by intraduodenal amino acid perfusion in man. *Gastroenterology*, 74:1261–1265.
33. Unger, R. H., and Eisentraut, A. M. (1969): Entero-insular axis. *Arch. Intern. Med.*, 123:261–266.
34. Verdonk, C. A., Rizza, R. A., Nelson, R. L., Go, V. L. W., Gerich, J. E., and Service, F. J. (1980): Interaction of fat-stimulated gastric inhibitory polypeptide on pancreatic alpha and beta cell function. *J. Clin. Invest.*, 65:1119–1125.

Insulin-like Growth Factors and Somatomedin

H. Ditschuneit and B. Pfeifle

Department of Internal Medicine II, University of Ulm, 7900 Ulm, Federal Republic of Germany

The topic of this chapter in honor of Professor Pfeiffer hardly deals with insulin-like growth factors and somatomedin. It is mostly by chance that these substances attract the interest of diabetologists and scientists involved in pancreative islets research. Nevertheless, there are two reasons why we have chosen to write on these topics. First of all, our engagement in these problems began more than 20 years ago, when we determined insulin-like activities in blood together with Professor Pfeiffer; second, the interest in insulin-like activities is being renewed today and might, perhaps soon, be shared by diabetologists.

During the first years of determining insulin-like activity, we repeatedly observed strikingly high levels of ILA in patients with atherosclerosis. ILA was found similarily elevated in maturity-onset diabetic patients, who are notorious for their high atherosclerotic morbidity. However, biological effects of "insulin" on isolated tissues were only partly due to insulin of pancreatic origin. The bulk of these effects was not inhibited by insulin antibodies. Therefore, these actions were called "atypical" or "nonsuppressible insulin-like activity (NSILA)" (5,18).

In our previous work, this insulin-like activity could not be assigned to just one protein fraction, but was rather distributed over several of the electrophoretically separated globuline bands. Acid-alcohol precipitation of serum proteins left insulin-like activity with the albumin-rich supernatant. This fraction, called "synalbumin" (21) even antagonizes insulin actions on the isolated diaphragm, thereby attracting the interest of many diabetologists some years ago. In our opinion, insulin-like activities of synalbumin appeared much more significant. We have spent much of our time with its isolation (2).

Meanwhile, the field of insulin-like serum fractions, which are not inhibited by insulin antibodies, has attracted broad interest from many of those engaged in metabolism research. Serum factors, which induce growth of cells in culture, were found to exhibit features of NSILA and, vice versa, NSILA showed growth-promoting activities. The number of these serum factors increases with years (Table 1). Reliable amino-acid analysis is lacking for most of these preparations. Therefore, it cannot be decided today whether or not these different substances only share common structures or whether or not there is a real difference.

Serum growth factors are also of great significance to the pathogenesis of atherosclerosis. According to Ross and Glomset (16,17), the atherosclerotic process originates from the proliferation of smooth muscle cells within the arterial wall. What triggers these cells to proliferate? Blood-born growth factors suggest themselves as the possible inducers of smooth muscle cell proliferation. Similarly, it might be highly possible that

TABLE 1

Nonsuppressible insulin-like activity (Froesch et al. (5))
   precipitated in acid-ethanol (NSILA-P)
   soluble in acid-ethanol (NSILA-S)
Atypical insulin (Samaan et al. (18))

Insulin-like growth factors (IGF) (Rinderknecht and Humble (15))
   IGF I (MW 7649)
   IGF II (MW 7471)

Sulfation factor, thymidin factor (19a)
Somatomedin (1a)
Somatomedin A (5a)
Somatomedin C (22a)
Multiplication stimulation activity (MSA) (14a)
Platelet-derived growth factor (PDGF) (17)
Epidermal growth factor (EGF) (1b)
Fibroblast growth factor (FGF) (6a)

these growth factors were somehow related to or even identical with factors with insulin-like activities and that, therefore, the increased levels of ILA in atherosclerotic patients might be of pathogenic significance for this degenerative blood vessel disease. Growth factors collected under the terms "somatomedin" or "insulin-like growth factors" are subject to regulation by growth hormone, whereas increasing growth hormone concentrations also elevate ILA. Concerning the possible interrelations of atherosclerosis and insulin-like growth factors, the following clinical observations might be important:

1. Dwarfs with isolated growth hormone deficiency and sharply decreased blood levels or lack of somatomedin or IGF never suffer from atherosclerosis, even when several of the well-known risk factors are present simultaneously (9).
2. Premature manifestation of atherosclerosis is observed in patients with increased growth hormone secretion as, for instance, in acromegaly. These patients also exhibit high blood levels of insulin-like growth factors.
3. Increased growth hormone and high ILA are a common feature of atherosclerotic patients (Fig. 1).
4. Similarly, increased ILA and growth hormone levels were observed in diabetic patients, who are notorious for their high incidence of atherosclerosis.

Insulin-like activity of human blood originates from two different fractions. The first one co-migrates with globulins in electrophoresis and is precipitated by alcoholic trichloracetic acid. The second fraction contributes to the albumin band and is not precipitated by acid-alcohol treatment of serum. It constitutes the minor part of total ILA found in whole serum. This soluble fraction, the NSILAs of Froesch and co-workers (10) can be separated from a carrier protein under acid conditions. Then, it shows insulin-like actions on muscle and fat.

According to Zapf et al. (25), the biological actions of this fraction is completely neutralized in serum by binding to the carrier protein. They claimed that only the globulin-bound ILA fractions were active in untreated serum. In our studies, this conclusion can only be drawn concerning the action on isolated

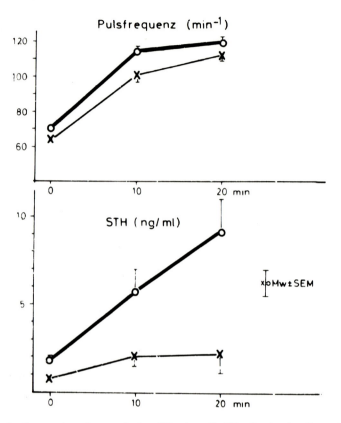

FIG. 1. Ergometer charge during 20 min with 32 atherosclerotic patients (o — o) and 14 normal control persons (× — ×). Effect on STH blood level and pulse rate.

muscle *in vitro*, but it does not hold true *in vivo*, when intraperitoneal injection is used (Figs. 2, 3). Under these conditions, nonsuppressible insulin effects can be detected on both muscle and fat, although the action on muscle tissue is considerably inferior to the effect on fat. Acid precipitation removes the globulin band with insulin-like activity *in vivo* as well as *in vitro* (Figs. 4, 5). In contrast, albumin-associated ILA can still be further observed, but no increase in its activity is presumably caused by separation from its carrier protein.

These results, obtained by intraperitoneal injection, certainly do not meet the conditions of intravascular blood stream. Nevertheless, they indicate that the active principal might be split

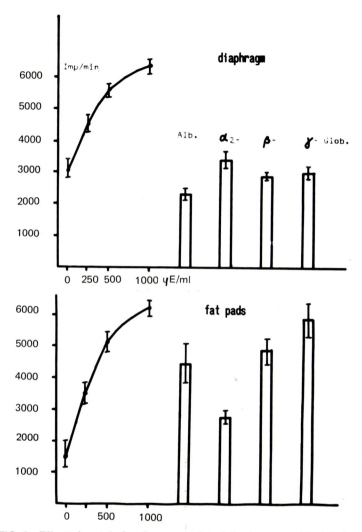

FIG. 2. Effect of protein fractions on isolated diaphragm and isolated epididymal fat pads. Incorporation of U-C^{14}-glucose into glycogen and lipids. Comparison with crist. insulin.

from a carrier protein under neutral conditions. Therefore, one might conclude that this fraction is potentially bioactive, reaching the target tissue via the blood stream.

Starting with 6 tons of serum protein, Rinderknecht and Humbel (15) succeeded in isolating two effective polypeptides from these albumin-associated ILAs, called IGF I and IGF II.

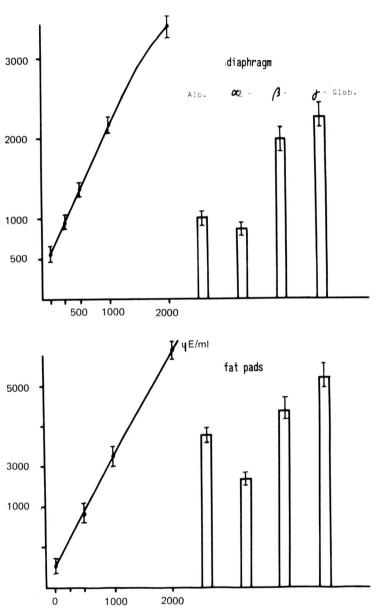

FIG. 3. Effect of protein fractions on diaphragm and epididymal fat pads following i.p. injection. Incorporation of U-C^{14}-glucose into glycogen and lipids. Comparison with crist. insulin.

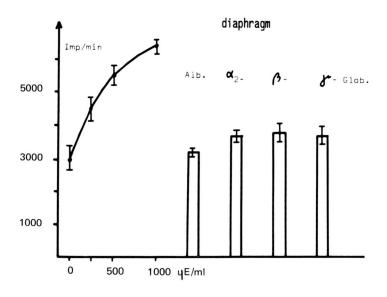

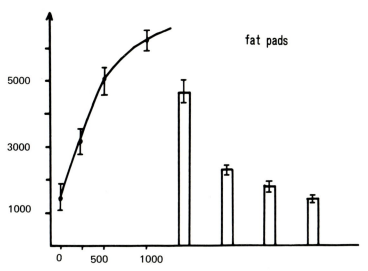

FIG. 4. Effect of supernatant of TCA-precipitated protein fractions on isolated diaphragm and isolated epididymal fat pads. Incorporation of U-C[14]-glucose into glycogen and lipids. Comparison with crist. insulin.

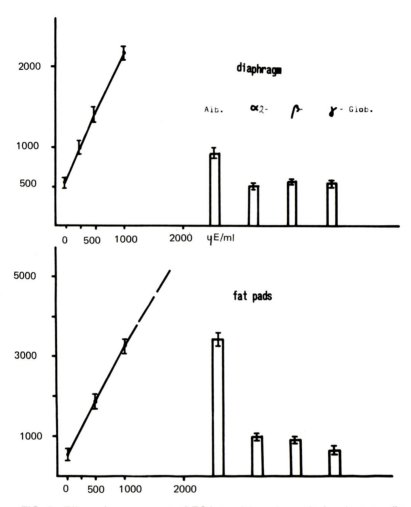

FIG. 5. Effect of supernatant of TCA-precipitated protein fractions on diaphragm and epididymal fat pads following i.p. injection. Incorporation of U-C^{14}-glucose into glycogen and lipids. Comparison with crist. insulin.

Amino-acid analysis of these polypeptides reveals striking similarities to proinsulin. Zapf et al. (23) therefore presumed that the three polypeptides—proinsulin, IGF I, and IGF II—would share one common phylogenetic origin. During evolution, approximately at the time of the first vertebrates on earth, some 600 million years ago, they might have descended from the same precursor. Insulin-like growth factor, which, unlike proinsulin, does not need to undergo proteolysis for activation, shows a closer affinity to the original protein.

Somatomedin C, which was detected in the investigation of somatotrophic hormone actions, is probably identical to IFG I (22). Both polypeptides exhibit biological insulin actions and mitogenic effects on cultured fibroblasts of rats and humans. They stimulate synthesis of DNA, RNA, protein, and cell proliferation. Binding competition studies revealed identical radioimmunological features. IGF affects embryonic chicken cartilage growth as much as somatomedin C. Serum concentrations of both IGF and sometomedin C are dependent on intact growth hormone secretion.

To clarify the significance of insulin-like growth factors to the pathogenesis of atherosclerosis, we performed similar studies by utilizing an *in vitro* system of cultured rat and human smooth muscle cells. Growth factors were isolated from several thousands of liters of serum. A direct comparison to IGF or somatomedin C presently is lacking because our polypeptide has not yet undergone amino-acid analysis so far. Therefore, our substance has been tentatively called "IGF Ulm." According to an analysis by Zapf in Zürich, the preparation contains IGF I and IGF II in a 3:1 ratio. There is no radioimunological evidence for contamination with insulin.

The preparation procedure of IGF Ulm is depicted in Fig. 6. This procedure shares the first steps with the isolation of IGF and somatomedin (12). Isoelectric focusing was chosen as the final step. Experiments with labeled IGF, which were kindly provided by the Zürich Group and which did as well as the radioimmunological analysis of our preparation, clarified that IGF I is the predominant constituent of our preparation.

GROWTH PROMOTING ACTIVITY ON SMOOTH MUSCLE CELLS OF SERA OBTAINED FROM DIFFERENT PATIENT GROUPS

These investigations were performed utilizing cultured human smooth muscle cells, derived from surgical specimens of arterial walls from 40-to-60-year-old patients. Smooth muscle

1 ↓
Acid ethanol extraction

2 ↓
Gelchromatography Sephadex G75

3 ↓
Gelchromatography Sephadex G50

4 ↓
preparative isoelectric focusing pH 3–9

FIG. 6. Purification procedure for insulin-like growth factors (IGF I and IGF II).

cells proliferating from the arterial explants after some 3 weeks were repeatedly subcultured (11,13,14). All studies were done in cells between the 4. and 6. passage. Growth-promoting activity was quantified by determination of thymidine incorporation into DNA. The effects on smooth muscle cell proliferation of the different sera tested correlated well with their growth hormone content (Fig. 7). Sera obtained from acromegalic patients containing 30.0 ng/ml growth hormone were most effective. Diabetic sera containing 7.3 ng/ml growth hormone were also significantly superior to normal control sera (3.2 ng/ml), whereas sera from hypophysectomized patients without detectible growth hormone concentrations were ineffective in the smooth muscle cell assay. Zapf et al. (24) and Heinrich et al. (7) reported IGF levels to be significantly increased in acromegalic patients and strikingly decreased in hypophysectomized individuals. Similar results concerning the somatomedin levels were obtained by Furlanetto et al. (6) and Clemmons et al. (1). Data on diabetic patients are currently incomplete. Presumably, their IGF levels should be increased compared to normal controls due to the elevated STH contents, which are much like the increased ILA.

These results indicate that even in whole serum there are

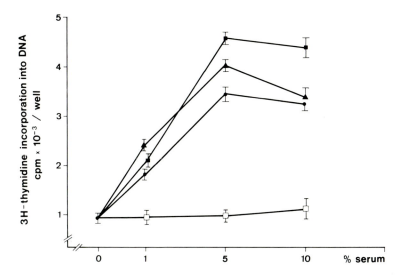

FIG. 7. Effect on DNS synthesis of serum of normal adults (●—●), and diabetic (▲—▲), acromegalic (■—■), and hypophysectomized (□—□) patients in human arterial smooth muscle cells.

growth factors affecting smooth muscle proliferation *in vitro*. Since these factors are presumably identical to IGF, IGF association to the carrier protein seems unlikely to abolish its growth-promoting effects, as claimed by Froesch and associates. Growth hormone itself lacks direct *in vitro* actions on smooth muscle cells. Therefore, different growth hormone concentrations of the sera used should not be contributed to the observed different effects.

BIOLOGICAL ACTIONS OF IGF ULM IN ISOLATED FAT CELLS AND CULTURED SMOOTH MUSCLE CELLS

In isolated fat cells, our IGF preparation (IGF Ulm) has insulin-like activity similar to the Zürich IGF. Following the incorporation of radio-labeled glucose into the lipid fraction of isolated rat fat cells, both preparations exhibited comparable activity. A specific activity of 9.9 mU/mg was calculated for the IGF Ulm as compared to insulin. IGF Zürich exhibited 8.5 mU/mg of insulin-like activity, which was not inhibited by insulin antibodies (Table 2). The stimulation of incorporation of (6-3H) thymidine into DNA of confluent-grown smooth muscle cells is shown in Fig. 8. Both factors stimulate this incorporation in a dose-dependent manner. A significant stimulating effect of both preparations is already observed at 10 ng/ml. Maximal stimulation occurs at 1 µg/ml with both factors. By using a medium containing 1% fetal calf serum, a more potent stimulation of (6-3H) thymidine incorporation could be observed in IGF from Zürich and in our isolated protein fraction.

Similar results were obtained from stimulation of (6-3H) uridine incorporation into RNA (Fig. 9) and stimulation of the protein synthesis (Fig. 10) by IGF of the Zürich group and by our protein fraction.

In all experiments our isolated protein fraction has a significantly higher effect than the Zürich preparation. A proportional comparison of both factors, insulin and 5% fetal calf serum, is shown in Table 3.

For the examination of the transport of amino acids into smooth muscle cells, experiments were done with 14 C-aminocyclopentane-carboxylic acid (Fig. 11). The IGF from Zürich and our isolated fraction were equipotent in concentrations up to 100.0 ng/ml. The effects of 100.0 ng/ml of both preparations correspond to the effect of 7.5% fetal calf serum.

TABLE 2

Addition		Stimulation of [^{14}C] incorporation into lipids of rat fat cells
Proteins	Amount	
	ng/ml	%
Control	0	0
IGF (Ulm)	1,000	3.8 ± 0.3
	10,000	7.9 ± 0.6
	100,000	11.6 ± 0.7
IGF (Zürich)	10,000	6.0 ± 0.4
Insulin	0.3	0.9 ± 0.3
	3	4.9 ± 0.7
	10	21.2 ± 1.3

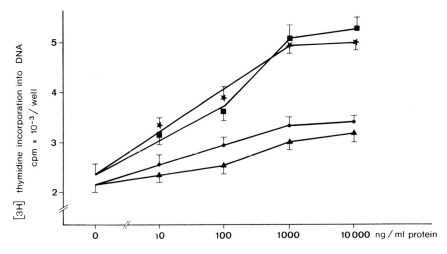

FIG. 8. DNA synthesis by IGF (Zürich) (▲—▲) (■—■) and IGF (Ulm) (●—●) (★—★) in cultivated arterial smooth muscle cells.

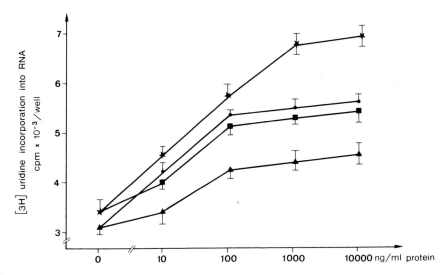

FIG. 9. RNA synthesis by IGF (Zürich) (▲—▲) (■—■) and IGF (Ulm) (●—●) (★—★) in cultivated arterial smooth muscle cells.

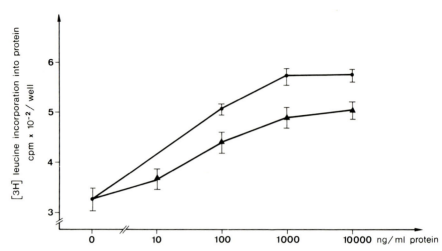

FIG. 10. Protein synthesis by IGF (Zürich) (▲—▲) and IGF (Ulm) (●—●) in cultivated arterial smooth muscle cells.

TABLE 3

Addition	Amount (ng/ml)	Stimulation of [3H]-thymidine incorporation into DNA (%)	Stimulation of [3H]-uridine incorporation into RNA (%)	Stimulation of [3H]-leucine incorporation into protein (%)
Control	0	0	0	0
IGF (Zürich)	100	19.4 ± 2.6	37.7 ± 2.9	33.3 ± 3.4
	1000	42.8 ± 3.2	47.5 ± 3.1	48.5 ± 3.3
IGF (Ulm)	100	38.3 ± 3.4	73.7 ± 5.6	53.0 ± 4.9
	1000	57.1 ± 4.2	80.3 ± 5.4	72.7 ± 5.9
Insulin	4000	15.1 ± 1.3	21.3 ± 1.7	18.7 ± 1.6
5% fetal calf serum	—	43.4 ± 3.3	40.9 ± 3.5	28.7 ± 2.7

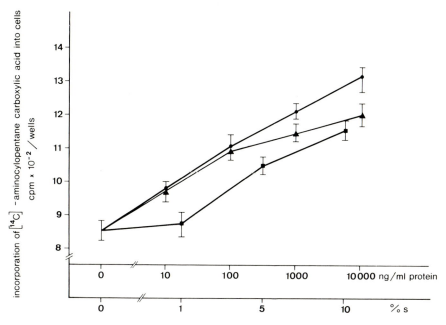

FIG. 11. Amino-acid transport into cultivated arterial smooth muscle cells by IGF (Zürich) (▲—▲) IGF (Ulm) (●—●), and fetal calf serum (■—■).

DEMONSTRATION OF SPECIFIC RECEPTORS FOR IGF ON CELL SURFACE OF CULTIVATED SMOOTH MUSCLE CELLS

In studies of competitive binding of radioactive-labeled IGF, specific receptors could be demonstrated. Specific binding of labeled IGF to the subcultures of confluently grown smooth muscle cells was 10%, calculated by subtracting nonspecific binding from total binding. Nonspecific binding was the binding of labeled IGF in the presence of 10 µg/ml unlabeled IGF. Half-maximal displacement of labeled IGF was achieved by 250 ng/ml of unlabeled IGF (Fig. 12). These experiments were done with labeled and unlabeled material from Zürich. With our fraction, the half-maximal displacement was reached with the higher concentrations of 1.2 µg/ml. Unlabeled proinsulin and insulin compete weakly with labeled IGF for its binding sites. Half-maximal displacement of labeled IGF is achieved by 6.3

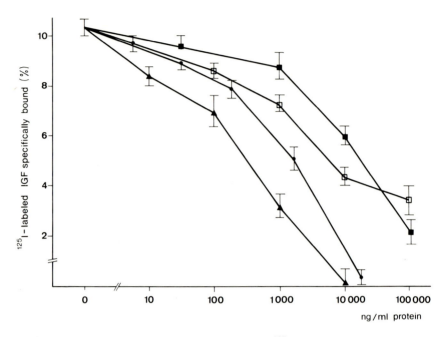

FIG. 12. Competitive inhibition of the binding of ^{125}I-labeled IGF by unlabeled IGF (Zürich) (▲—▲), IGF (Ulm) (●—●), proinsulin (□—□), and insulin (■—■) in cultured arterial smooth muscle cells.

μg/ml of unlabeled proinsulin and by 17.8 μg/ml of unlabeled insulin.

In studies with fibroblasts of chicken embryo, Zapf et al. (24) found a specific binding of only 0.3% to 0.9% at 30°C and 90 min of incubation. In isolated fat cells, the specific binding reached only 0.22% at 37°C and 45 min (19), whereas in the liver plasma membranes, a specific binding of IGF of approximately 14% at 20°C and 90 min could be demonstrated (8). If we compare these results with our findings at smooth muscle cells, we can conclude that smooth muscle cells are very sensitive to IGF and small amounts in the range of physiologic concentrations can stimulate their proliferation already.

The specific receptors for IGF and insulin, however, will be changed significantly by growth. This effect of growth was demonstrated at smooth muscle cells of different ages. For these studies the cells were plated to a density of 10^5 cells/ml. In culture medium containing 10% fetal calf serum, they reached confluency 3 days after the plating. On the fourth day, their growth was arrested. The results of the competitive binding experiments at different days of culture with labeled and unlabeled IGF and insulin are presented in Figs. 13 and 14. IGF competed with ^{125}I-IGF for its binding sites for the entire time of the experiment. Half-maximal inhibition of ^{125}I-IGF to unlabeled IGF varied with the growth status of the cell between 10 and 100 nmol/l. Insulin competed also with ^{125}I-IGF for its binding sites, but the displacement of ^{125}I-IGF from its binding sites by insulin varied significantly with the growth status of the cells. During the first 2 days, insulin competed only weakly with the labeled IGF for the binding sites. A significant inhibition of labeled IGF binding was produced by insulin only at high concentrations of 1 to 10 µmol/l. If the cells had reached confluency but growth had not yet been arrested, insulin would not have been able to displace IGF from its binding sites (see Fig. 13 C). However, the last 2 days when growth of the cells had been arrested, insulin inhibited binding of ^{125}I-IGF (see Fig. 13 d, e). The half-maximal displacement of IGF was reached at 1 umol/l (see Fig. 13 e).

These changes in competitive binding of IGF and insulin are presumably produced by changes of the IGF receptor and down regulation of the receptors for insulin. When, on the contrary, labeled insulin is bound to the cells, then insulin produced a half-maximal inhibition on the second and third day of culture at concentrations between 0.3 and 0.8 nmol/l (see Fig. 14 b, c). But when growth of the cells had been arrested, insulin was no longer able to displace ^{125}I-insulin from its binding sites (see Fig. 14, d, e). On the other hand, IGF competed with the labeled insulin for its binding sites over the whole term of our experiments. But the inhibition of the ^{125}I-insulin binding by IGF showed variations. In the first 2 days, IGF competed only weakly. During the last 2 days in culture, when growth had been arrested, the half-maximal inhibition of labeled insulin by IGF increased to 10 nmol/l (see Fig. 14 e).

These observations corroborate the hypothesis that growth effects are mediated by the IGF receptor, and metabolic effects are mediated by the insulin receptor. The same regulations for

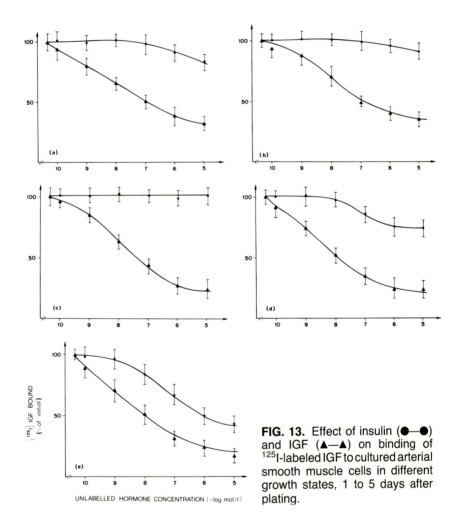

FIG. 13. Effect of insulin (●—●) and IGF (▲—▲) on binding of ^{125}I-labeled IGF to cultured arterial smooth muscle cells in different growth states, 1 to 5 days after plating.

ILGF AND SOMATOMEDIN 87

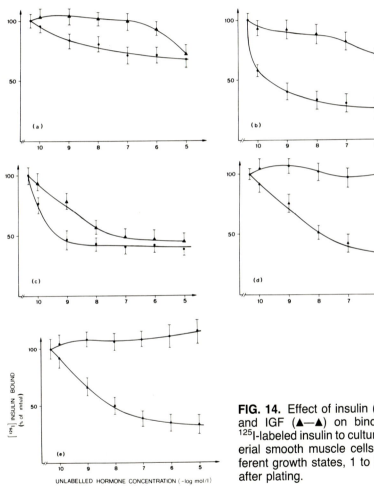

FIG. 14. Effect of insulin (●—●) and IGF (▲—▲) on binding of ^{125}I-labeled insulin to cultured arterial smooth muscle cells in different growth states, 1 to 5 days after plating.

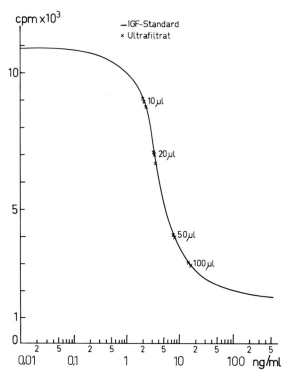

FIG. 15. Competitive dose response curve for the serum standard by radioimmunoassay.

the insulin receptor were described by Thomopoulos et al. (20) for cultured fibroblasts. All observations indicate that, with the change from growing state to stationary state, a modification of the IGF binding sites appeared. Therefore, insulin could now be bound to the IGF binding sites and was now able to compete with labeled IGF for its binding sites. IGF was now also able to inhibit labeled insulin binding. In the stationary state of the cells, insulin could not displace ^{125}I-insulin binding. This indicates the disappearance of specific insulin binding sites. We assume a down regulation of the binding sites by serum factors. The insulin action may now occur predominantly via IGF binding sites.

CONCLUSION

From clinical observations and our experimental results, we conclude that insulin-like growth factors may significantly contribute to the pathogenesis of atherosclerosis. Their potent growth-promoting effects are comparable only to those of the platelet-derived growth factor. There is no experimental evidence today that proves one group more effective in stimulating the proliferation of smooth muscle cells following an endothelial lesion or the insulin-like or platelet-derived growth factor. It is hoped that this question will be enlightened by further clinical studies correlating radioimmunologically determined IGF levels with the degree of atherosclerosis. An appropriate radioimmunoassay has been developed in our laboratory (Fig. 15). Its sensitivity and reproducibility are sufficient to allow reliable determination of serum amounts as small as 100 µl. The additional question of how the insulin-like growth factor isolated in our laboratory is related to IGF I or somatomedin C awaits further clearing by amino-acid analysis. This requires much more of the purified preparation, forcing us to extract again tons of serum. We might report on these forthcoming events by the time of the next birthday anniversary of Dr. Ernst Pfeiffer, when he has terminated another successful and healthy ten years.

REFERENCES

1. Clemmons, D. R., Van Wyk, J. J., Ridgway, E. C., Kliman, B., Kjellberg, R. N., and Underwood, L. E. (1979): Evaluation of acromegaly by radioimmunoassay of somatomedin C. *N. Engl. J. Med.*, 301:1138.
1a. Daughaday, W. H., Hall, K., Raben, M. S., Salomon, W. D., Van der Brande, L. I., Van Wyk, I. I. (1972): Somatomedin: Proposed designation for sulfation factor. *Nature*, 235:107.
1b. Cohen, S., Taylor, I. M. (1974): Epidermal growth factor: Chemical and biological characterization. *Recent Prog. Horm. Res.*, 30:533.
2. Ditschuneit, H. (1969): Definition and criteria of prediabetes. In: *Diabetes*, edited by J. Östman, pp. 479–485. Excerpta Medica Foundation, Amsterdam.
3. Östman, J., and Milner, R. D. G. (1969): In: *Diabetes*, p. 479. Excerpta Medica Foundation, Amsterdam.
4. Ditschuneit, H., Ditschuneit, H. H., Küter, E., Rakow, D., and Klör, H. U. (1974): The influence of exercise on growth hormone (STH)—secretion in males with atherosclerotic lesions. In: *Atherosclerosis IV*, edited by G. Schettler and A. Wetzel, p. 617. Springer-Verlag, Berlin, Heidelberg, New York.

5. Froesch, E. R., Burgi, H., Ramseier, E. B., Bally, P., and Labhart, A. J. (1963): Antibody suppressible and insulinlike activities in human serum and their physiologic significance. *J. Clin. Invest*, 42:1816.
5a. Fryklund, L., Skuttner, A., Sievertsson, H., Hall, K. (1976): Somatomedins A and B. Isolation, chemistry and *in vitro* effects. In: *Growth hormone and related peptides*, edited by A. Pecile and E. E. Muller, pp. 156–168. Experta Medica, Amsterdam.
6. Furlanetto, R. W., Underwood, L. E., Van Wyk, J. J., and D'Ercole, A. J. (1977): Estimation of somatomedin C levels in normals and patients with pituitary disease by radioimmunoassay. *J. Clin. Invest.*, 60:648.
6a. Gospodarowicz. G. (1975): Purification of a fibroblast growth factor from bovine pituitary. *I. Biol. Chem.*, 250:2515.
7. Heinrich, U., Schalch, D. S., Koch, J. G., and Johnson, C. J. (1978): Nonsuppressible insulin-like activity (NSILA). *J. Clin. Endocrinol. Metab.*, 46:672.
8. Megyesi, K., Kahn, C. R., Roth, J., Neville, D. M., Nissley, S. P., Humbel, R. E., and Froesch, E. R. (1975): The NSILA-s-receptor in liver plasma membranes—characterization and comparison with the insulin receptor. *J. Biol. Chem.*, 250:8990.
9. Merimee, T. J. (1972): Comparative clinical and metabolic studies in diabetes mellitus and sexual ateliotic dwarfism. *Isr. J. Med. Sci.*, 8:420.
10. Oelz, O., Froesch, E. R., Bünzli, H. F., Humbel, R. E., and Ritschard, W. J. (1972–1976): Antibody—suppressible and nonsuppressible insulin-like activities. In: *Handbuch Physiology*, Sect. 7, Endocrinology, 1:685.
11. Pfeifle, B., and Ditschuneit, H. (1983): Two separate receptors for insulin and insulin-like growth factors on arterial smooth muscle cells. *Endokrinologie*, 81:280.
12. Pfeifle, B., and Ditschuneit, H. (1980); The effect of insulin and insulin-like growth factors on cell proliferation of human smooth muscle cells. *Artery*, 8:336.
13. Pfeifle, B., Ditschuneit, H. H., and Ditschuneit, H. (1982): Binding and biological actions of insulin-like growth factors on human arterial smooth muscle cells. *Horm. Metab. Res.*, 8:409.
14. Pfeifle, B., and Ditschuneit, H. (1983): Receptors for insulin-like growth factors in cultured arterial smooth muscle cells depend on their growth state. *J. Endocr.*, 96:251.
14a. Pierson, R. W., Temin, H. M. (1972): The partial purification from calf-serum of a fraction with multiplication stimulating activity for chicken fibroblasts in cell culture and with non-suppressible insulin-like activity. *I. Cell Physiol.*, 79:319.
15. Rinderknecht, E., and Humbel, R. E. (1976): Polypeptides with non-suppressible insulin-like and cell-growth promoting activities in human serum: isolation, chemical characterization and some biological properties of terms I and II. *Proc. Natl. Acad. Sci. USA*, 73:2365.
16. Ross, R. W., and Glomset, J. (1973): Atherosclerosis and the arterial smooth muscle cell. *Science*, 180:1332.
17. Ross, R., Glomset, J., Kariya, B., and Harker, L. (1974): A platelet dependent serum factor that stimulates the proliferation of arterial smooth muscle cells in vitro. *Proc. Natl. Acad. Sci. USA*, 71:1207.

18. Samaan, N. A., Dempster, W. J., Fraser, R., Please, N. W., and Stillma, D. J. (1962): Further immunological studies on the term of circulating insulin. *J. Endocrinol.*, 24:263.
19. Schoenle, E., Zapf, J., and Froesch, E. R. (1977): Effect of insulin and NSILA on adipocytes of normal and diabetic rats: receptor binding, glucose transport and glucose metabolism. *Diabetologica*, 13:243.
19a. Salomon, W. D., Daughaday, W. H. (1957): A hormonally controlled serum facor which stimulates incorporation by cartilage *in vitro*. *I. Lab. Clin. Med.*, 49:825.
20. Thomopoulos, P., Willingham, M. C., and Pastan, M. (1978): Studies on the regulation of insulin receptors in cultured BALB/3 T 3 fibroblasts. *Exp. Cell Res.*, 116:478.
21. Vallance-Owen, J., Drumes, E., and Campbell, P. N. (1958): Insulin antagonism in plasma of diabetic patients and normal subjects. *Lancet*, 2:336.
22. Van Wyk, J. J., Swobody, M. E., and Underwood, L. E. (1980): Evidence from radio ligand assays that somatomedin C and insulinlike growth factor are similar to each other and different from other somatomedin. *J. Clin. Endocrinol. Metab.*, 50:206.
22a. Van Wyk, I. I., Underwood, L. E., Hintz, R. L., Clemmons R. B., Voina, S. I., Wearer, R. P. (1974): The somatomedins: A family of insulin-like hormones under growth hormone control. *Recent Prog. Horm. Res.*, 30:259.
23. Zapf, J., Froesch, E. R., and Humbel, R. E. (1981): The insulin-like growth factors (IGF) of human serum: chemical and biological characterization and aspects of their possible physiological role. *Current Top. Cell Regul.*, 19:257.
24. Zapf, J., Mäder, M., Waldvogel, M., Schlach, D. S., Froesch, E. R. (1975): Specific binding of nonsuppressible insulin-like activity to chicken embryo fibroblasts and to a solubilized fibroblast receptor. *Arch. Biochem. Biophys.*, 168:630.
25. Zapf, J., Schoenle, E., Jagars, G., Sand, I., Grünwald, J., and Froesch, E. R. (1979): Inhibition of the action of nonsuppressible insulin-like activity on isolated rat fat cells by binding to its carrier proteins. *J. Clin. Invest.*, 63:1077.

The Importance of Islets of Langerhans for Modern Endocrinology, edited by K. Federlin and J. Scholtholt, Raven Press, New York © 1984.

Pathomorphology of the Pancreas in Diabetes

W. Gepts

Department of Pathology, Fak. Geneeskunde & Farmacie, Vrije Universiteit Brussel, Brussels, Belgium

The etiology of the most common types of human diabetes remains unknown; they are therefore designated as primary or idiopathic. Other much rarer cases result either from a destructive process involving the pancreas as a whole (e.g., pancreatitis, hemochromatosis, cancer) or from extrapancreatic factors (e.g., peripheral resistance to insulin, excessive secretion of hormonal antagonists to insulin). They are grouped under the name of secondary diabetes.

Despite the fact that heterogeneity of diabetes has become more evident in recent years, its pancreatic pathology is still represented by two distinct entities, roughly corresponding to the classic juvenile-onset and maturity-onset types of the disease. It has been argued that classification by age at onset is inappropriate because both insulin-dependent and noninsulin-dependent diabetes can occur at any age. It has been emphasized also that the pattern of inheritance is correlated not with age at onset, but with the clinical type of diabetes (48). Indeed, there are cases of late-onset, insulin-dependent, and ketosis-prone diabetes with a pancreatic pathology resembling that of classical juvenile diabetes (31). Likewise, young subjects may occasionally develop a mild type of diabetes with only minor and nonspecific changes in the pancreas. However, such cases are rare. In most maturity-onset diabetic subjects, including many genuine insulin-dependent cases, the pancreatic pathology is distinctly different from that of juvenile-onset cases, both quantitatively and qualitatively.

PANCREATIC MORPHOPATHOLOGY IN MATURITY-ONSET DIABETES

Maturity-onset diabetes is usually a mild type of the disease, often associated with obesity. Biologically, it is characterized by retention of endogenous insulin secretion, although with altered secretory dynamics; the absence of ketosis; and insulin resistance due to diminished target cell response to insulin (56). The whole range of insulin responses to glucose, from low to supranormal, has been reported in patients with maturity-onset diabetes. There has been considerable controversy about the parts played by B-cell dysfunction and by insulin resistance in this type of diabetes (13,14,58). Obviously, there is a spectrum of subtypes of noninsulin-dependent diabetes. It is not surprising, therefore, that in this type of the disease the pancreatic pathology is extremely variable.

Changes in the Pancreas as a Whole

There are no specific gross changes in the pancreas of maturity-onset diabetic subjects. In late-onset diabetes the weight of the pancreas is usually within normal range (15,30). Fatty infiltration and fibrosis are common in the pancreas of elderly diabetic subjects, but not any more so than in nondiabetic subjects of corresponding age.

Volume of Islet Tissue

Using crude methods, many investigators have estimated the total volume of islet tissue. Their unanimous conclusion that the total volume of endocrine tissue is usually reduced in cases of maturity-onset diabetes has been confirmed by a recent study performed with immunocytochemical staining techniques and precise stereological methods (51a). However, the reduction is moderate and a large overlap exists between the figures observed in diabetic and in nondiabetic subjects.

General Appearance of the Islets

There are no distinct differences in the general appearance of the islets between maturity-onset diabetic subjects and aging nondiabetic subjects. In both, the islets have lost the compact structure characteristic of the islets in healthy young subjects. To a greater or lesser extent, they have become subdivided in lobules by thin fibrous septa enclosing the capillaries. The center of the lobules is occupied by B cells; the A cells are usually aligned along the fibrovascular septa (Fig. 1). The D cells have a more haphazard arrangement (26).

Fibrosis

Fibrosis of the islets is the most common lesion in the islets of elderly diabetic subjects, but also the least specific, being found as well in the islets of many nondiabetic subjects of the same age. It is often associated with some degree of pancreatic fibrosis and may be partly related to parenchymal sclerosis of vascular origin (20).

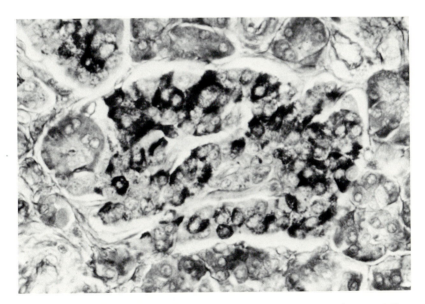

FIG. 1. Islet in the pancreas of a noninsulin-dependent, maturity-onset diabetic. Note the fibrous septa and the well-granulated B cells (*dark cells*). Aldehyde thionine staining. × 504.

Islet Hyalinosis (Amyloidosis)

Islet hyalinosis (Fig. 2) is often found in the islets of maturity-onset diabetic subjects. In the literature the frequency of its occurrence is usually rated at 40% (62), but its incidence increases with age; it is found in more than 50% of the diabetic subjects over the age of 50 (27). Westermark and Wilander (64) recently reported that they have been able to detect hyalin deposits in the islets of every maturity-onset diabetic subject. Islet hyalinosis should actually be better designated as amyloidosis because the hyalin substance has all the staining and ultrastructural characteristics of amyloid. Amyloidosis of the islets is not diagnostic of diabetes because it is found also in nondiabetic patients, albeit much more rarely and to a lesser degree (6). However, the frequency of hyaline islets is so much greater in maturity-onset diabetic than in nondiabetic subjects of corresponding age that there can be little doubt that this lesion is in

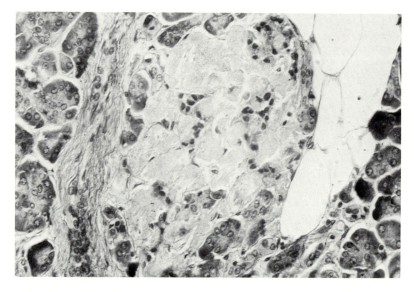

FIG. 2. Islet hyalinosis (amyloidosis) in a pancreatic islet of a maturity-onset diabetic subject. Gomori's chromium hematoxylin phloxine. × 315.

some way related to the diabetic state (7). Nevertheless, the exact nature of this relationship remains obscure.

Cellular Composition of the Islets

Numerous studies of the cellular composition of the islets in maturity-onset diabetes have been performed, most often with staining techniques of limited specificity and sensitivity. All of these studies reached the same conclusion that the proportion of B cells versus non-B cells is reduced in this type of diabetes (55). However, a considerable overlap between the figures of the diabetic and nondiabetic groups was observed. Moreover, all these studies were performed with staining techniques that did not allow one to distinguish between the different types of non-B cells, and before Orci and associates demonstrated the heterogeneity of islet cell type distribution within the pancreas (43). Taking into account this new anatomical knowledge and using specific immunocytochemical staining of the four principal islet cell types and painstaking stereological methods, Rahier (51a) has recently been able to confirm the relative preponderance of non-B cells versus B cells in the pancreas of maturity-onset diabetic subjects. This preponderance results from both a slight decrease of the total amount of B cells and an increased amount of A cells.

Changes in the B Cells

Considering the diabetic state of the patients, the B cells of subjects with a maturity-onset type of diabetes show surprisingly few changes. Hydropic appearance is rare. Even in untreated diabetic subjects with fasting hyperglycemia, the B cells are often small and show little or no degranulation. Bell (5) observed degranulation of the B cells in all diabetic patients under the age of 20, but in only 34% of those over 60 years of age. A significant decrease in the nuclear size of the B cells of elderly diabetic subjects was demonstrated by Westermark and Grimelius (63). A reduction in size of the Golgi apparatus and a lesser development of the endoplasmic reticulum were reported by Kawanishi et al. (26) in electron microscopic studies of the B cells in cases of maturity-onset diabetes. These observations strongly suggest a reduced functional activity of the B cells in many elderly diabetic subjects, a paradoxical finding in view of the chronic hyperglycemic state of these patients. The exact site of the functional deficiency of the B cells in many cases of maturity-onset diabetes remains obscure.

PANCREATIC MORPHOPATHOLOGY IN JUVENILE-ONSET DIABETES

Juvenile-onset diabetes is usually a severe, insulin-dependent, and ketosis-prone type of diabetes, developing in a lean person. Biologically, it is characterized by a total or almost total loss of endogenous insulin secretion. In this type of diabetes and in striking contrast to maturity-onset diabetes, the islets of Langerhans show severe and pathognomonic changes. These changes represent an adequate basis for the observed physio-pathological phenomena. They have also been instrumental in tackling the problem of the etiology of this type of diabetes.

Changes in the Pancreas as a Whole

In early-onset, insulin-dependent diabetes, the pancreas is often much smaller than normal. This reduction appears to result either from a secondary atrophy or from an arrest of growth because at the onset of the disease, the weight of the organ is normal. Rahier (51) has made the interesting observation that this secondary atrophy affects only the PP-cells-poor part of the pancreas but spares the PP-cells-rich part. In the pancreas of subjects with long-standing diabetes, the PP-cells-rich lobe therefore represents a higher percentage of the total pancreatic volume (between 16.5% and 26.5%) than in the normal pancreas in which it does not exceed 11%.

General Appearance of the Islets

The general appearance of the islets of Langerhans in insulin-dependent juvenile diabetes always show distinctive and characteristic changes. Already at clinical onset, the majority of these islets are small and so unobtrusive that they easily escape detection in routinely stained sections. These islets are composed of thin cords of small cells (Fig. 3) arranged in a more or less abundant fibrous stroma (26). In the past these islets have been regarded as atrophic, but with the newer and more sensitive immunocytochemical techniques, they have been shown to consist of approximately two-thirds glucagon cells and the remaining third somatostatin cells (28,42). As a rule, these pseudoatrophic islets do not contain B cells.

Another much rarer type of islets is found in the pancreas of young diabetic subjects, but only in those who have died after a disease of short duration (16,19). They occur only in localized areas of the pancreas. They are quite variable in size, some very small, some large and even hypertrophic (Fig. 4). They are composed mainly of B cells showing signs of a tremendous functional hyperactivity, such as large vesicular nuclei, degranulation, and increased RNA-content of the cytoplasm. In addition to the B cells, these islets also contain a small proportion of well-granulated A and D cells.

In cases of long-standing, insulin-dependent juvenile diabetes, a third type of islets is often prominent (18). These islets are

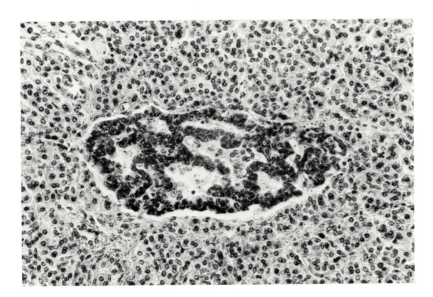

FIG. 3. Pseudoatrophic islet in the pancreas of an insulin-dependent young diabetic subject. Mallory's phosphotungstic hematoxylin. × 184.5.

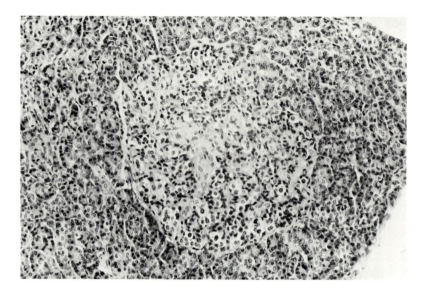

FIG. 4. Large, hyperactive islet with hydropic change of B cells in a young, recent-onset, insulin-dependent subject. Mallory's phosphotungstic hematoxylin. × 118.

composed of cords of cylindrical cells, arranged in a serpentine pattern, and often apparently arising from the epithelium of medium-sized ducts (Fig. 5). Such islets were already admirably described by MacCallum (36) as hypertrophic islands characteristic of the diabetic pancreas. They were completely disregarded later on, probably because of their failure to stain with any of the older granule staining techniques. It has been demonstrated that in juvenile diabetic subjects, such islets are almost entirely composed of cells containing "pancreatic polypeptide" (PP). Orci and associates (2,38,43,45) have pointed out that islets of this type occur in the dorsal part of the head of the pancreas of normal subjects, in whom, in addition to PP cells, a smaller proportion of B and D cells and rare A cells are contained. On the basis of routine necropsy specimens, my group has described hyperplasia of PP cells in the pancreas of patients with long-standing, insulin-dependent diabetes (18). In a recent study performed with rigorous stereological methods on adequately sampled pancreas from four insulin-dependent diabetics,

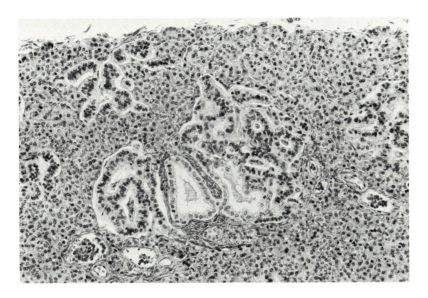

FIG. 5. PP islet composed of cords of cylindrical cells arranged in a serpentine pattern and connected to ductal epithelium. Mallory's phosphotungstic hematoxylin. × 118.

Rahier (*unpublished personal communication*, 1982) found total amounts of PP cells similar to control values in three cases, and a markedly elevated amount of PP cells in one case.

Quantitative Changes of the Islet Cells

As already mentioned, the majority of the islets in the pancreas of juvenile-onset diabetic subjects are small and composed only of A and D cells. Therefore, it is not surprising that, even in recent-onset cases, the estimated number of B cells is already reduced to 10% of normal or less (16,28). Until recently, it was generally assumed that in most cases of juvenile-onset diabetes, insulin secretion disappears completely within a short time after the time of diagnosis. This view was based on studies with conventional staining techniques in which it was stated that B cells could no longer be detected after a clinical duration of the disease longer than 1 year. However, the application of new, more sensitive techniques has revealed that B cells can still be detected, albeit in very low number, in 50% of the diabetic subjects who have had the disease for less than 10 years and in 18% of those with the disease of longer duration (28). These findings correlate well with clinical studies of C-peptide secretion, demonstrating a residual insulin secretion in some juvenile-onset diabetic subjects many years after the onset of their disease (4,9,23). Contrary to the B cells, the A, D, and PP cells remain present in large number throughout the course of the disease (28,41).

Distortion of Islet Architecture

Another important contribution of the modern immunocytochemical methods is the demonstration of the profound distortion of the structural organization of the islets. Not only have the B cells disappeared from all or from nearly all the islets, but, especially in cases of long duration, many A and D cells, and even some of the surviving B cells, are no longer contained within islets; they are irregularly scattered as single cells (Fig. 6) in the exocrine tissue (28). In view of Orci and Unger's concept (41,44,59) of the possible importance of intraislet paracrine relationship among islet cells, it is tempting to speculate that the abnormal secretory behavior of the A cells in juvenile-onset diabetes results from the loss of normal contacts with B and D cells.

Mechanisms of B Cell Destruction in Juvenile-Onset Diabetes—Insulitis

The mechanisms of the selective destruction of the B cells in juvenile-onset diabetes have not been convincingly elucidated. Pathomorphologic observations strongly suggest that, at least in part of the cases, the B cells are destroyed by an inflammatory process, insulitis, that has been going on without notice during the preclinical phase of the disease. This suggestion is in keeping with reports that islet cell antibodies (ICA), now widely accepted as markers of islet damage, may appear months or even years before the clinical onset of diabetes (8,22,53).

Insulitis characteristically appears as an infiltration of some, never of all, the islets by lymphocytes (Fig. 7). The cellular infiltrate is sharply limited to the islets. In some cases it is

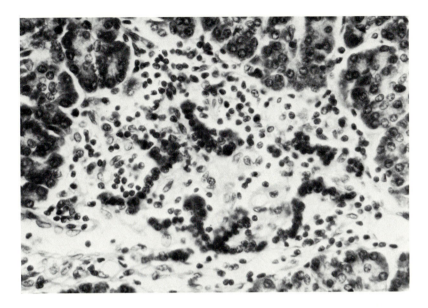

FIG. 6. Glucagon cells (*black*) scattered in the exocrine tissue. Long-standing, juvenile-onset diabetes. Immunoperoxidase staining method of Sternberger. × 237.5.

localized at their periphery, in others it extends into the islets and profoundly disrupts their architecture.

The reports about the frequency of insulitis are still conflicting. Maclean and Ogilvie (37) found it in only 3 of their 18 acute cases. Doniach and Morgan (12) did not find it at all in any of their 13 recent-onset cases. I observed it in 16 of 23 young insulin-dependent diabetic subjects examined within 6 months of the first symptoms of diabetes (26,28). Junker et al. (25) noticed it in 6 of 11 young diabetics who had died within 2 months of onset of diabetes.

Several explanations can be offered for these discrepant reports. In most of the cases, insulitis affects only a few islets and is discrete; it may therefore easily escape detection. Insulitis is an elusive lesion; it has never been found after a duration of disease exceeding 1 or 2 years. Junker et al (25) have suggested that the age at onset of diabetes may be of importance. Indeed, 49% of

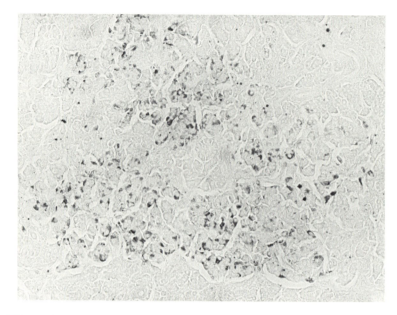

FIG. 7. Lymphocytic infiltration in an islet of a young, recent-onset, insulin-dependent diabetic subject. Gomori's chromium hematoxylin. × 315.

the cases reported in the literature had become diabetic before the age of 10, and 95% before the age of 20. Only two well-documented cases have been described in insulin-dependent diabetic subjects with onset of disease in old age (31). The cytological composition of the islets also plays a role in determining the presence of lymphocytic infiltration; morphologic observations strongly suggest that lymphocytes involved in insulitis are attracted selectively by islets that still contain B cells (28), and such islets have become rare at the time of clinical onset of insulin-dependent diabetes.

The presence of a lymphocytic infiltration in the islets of young recent-onset, insulin-dependent diabetics is compatible with an autoimmune process, with a previous viral infection, or with a combination of the two. Rare cases have been described in which a virus seems to have been directly responsible for the B-cell damage. In the few cases that have come to autopsy

(21,65), the islets were still numerous and showed conspicuous insulitis. Many B cells were still present, but they showed evidence of severe damage. Islet cell damage has recently been described in 28 of 250 children with fatal viral infection, but without clinical evidence of diabetes (24). However, insulitis has also been observed in the pancreatic islets of patients with a polyendocrine autoimmune disease.

Insulitis is known to occur spontaneously in animals: cattle (3,11,46,47), cat (17), BB/W rats (34,35,40,54), NZO mice (28). It has also been induced in laboratory animals by a variety of experimental procedures: active immunization against homologous or heterologous insulin, injection of anti-insulin serum; injection of pancreatic or islet tissue; inoculation of viruses; the multiple subdiabetogenic dose streptozotocin model (for a review, see ref. 32). Evidence is accumulating that in all these models, including the experimental viral model, cell-mediated autoimmunity is involved. The latest evidence available suggests that cellular immune reactions against pancreatic islet cells may emerge from a dysregulation of the immune system, which may be induced by a variety of factors (29).

The morphological evidence that lymphocytes could be the agents for B-cell destruction does not rule out other possible mechanisms. Cases of rodenticide-induced, insulin-dependent diabetes have been described (39,49,50). There has been a recent report (10) on four patients who developed type I diabetes after being treated with pentamidine for a Pneumocystis carinii pneumonia.

The recent suggestion (57) that B cell destruction may result from cumulative insults by virus and chemicals, either directly or through the mediation of immunopathological reactions, on a background of a genetic predisposition, is also worthy of consideration. This suggestion receives support from the observation that pseudoatrophic islets, mainly composed of glucagon cells without B cells, which are the hallmark of a previously inflicted damage, can be detected in seemingly acute, viral-induced diabetes (*personal observation, unpublished*).

In his introduction to the first edition of *Volk* and the late Wellman's book, *The Diabetic Pancreas* (33), Rachmiel Levine pointed out "that research direction in diabetes has never proceeded in a straight line. Observations were frequently made which went unnoticed and unsung and had to be rediscovered at a more propitious time."

Pathomorphological studies of the diabetic pancreas offers many examples of such erratic movements. It is my firm belief that much can still be learned from looking at the pancreas of diabetic subjects, especially if newly available techniques and methods are applied whenever possible and if the findings are interpreted not only from a pure morphological point of view, but in close conjunction with clinicians and research workers.

ACKNOWLEDGMENTS

Part of the work included in this chapter was supported by grants from the Belgian "Fonds voor Geneeskundig Wetenschappelijk Onderzoek" (3.0023.78 en 3.0024.82), from the "Nationale Bank van België," and from the Belgian "Ministerie voor Wetenschapsbeleid" (80-85/9). The excellent assistance of N. Beulens and S. Pieters is gratefully acknowledged.

REFERENCES

1. Appel, M. C., Rossini, A. A., Williams, R. M., and Like, A. A. (1978): Viral studies in streptozotocin-induced pancreatic insulitis. *Diabetologia*, 15:327–336.
2. Baetens, D., Malaisse-Lagae, F., Perrelet, A., and Orci, L. (1979): Endocrine pancreas: three dimensional reconstruction shows two types of islets of Langerhans. *Nature*, 206:1323–1325.
3. Barboni, E. and Manocchio, I. (1962): Alterazionia pancreatiche con diabete mellito post-aftoso. *Arch. Vet. Stal.*, 13:477–489.
4. Beischer, W., Raptis, R., Keller, L., Heinze, E., Schröder, K. E., and Pfeiffer, E. F. (1975): Characterization of residual beta-cell function in diabetes by a new C-peptide radioimmunoassay (abstract). *Diabetologia*, 11:332.
5. Bell, E. T. (1953): Significance of degranulation in the islets of Langerhans in diabetes mellitus. *Diabetes*, 2:125–129.
6. Bell, E. T. (1959): Hyalinization of the islets of Langerhans in nondiabetic individuals. *Am. J. Path.*, 35:801–805.
7. Bell, E. T. (1960): *Diabetes Mellitus. A clinical and pathological study of 2529 cases*, edited Charles C Thomas Publisher, pp. 51–55. Springfield, Illinois.
8. Betterle, C., Lanette, F., Tiengo, A., and Trevisan, A. (1982): Letter to the Editor. *Lancet*, 1:284–285.
9. Block, M. B., Rosenfield, R. L., Mako, M. E., Steiner, D. F., and Rubenstein, A. K. (1973): Sequential changes in beta-cell function in

insulin-treated diabetic patients assessed by C-peptide immunoreactivity. *N. Engl. J. Med.*, 288:1144–1148.
10. Bouchard, P., Sai, P., Reach, G., Caubarière, I., Ganeval, D., and Assan, R. (1982): Diabetes mellitus following Pentamidine-induced hypoglycemia in humans. *Diabetes*, 31:40–45.
11. Christensen, N. O., and Schambye, P. (1930): On diabetes mellitus hos kvaeg. *Nord. Vet. Med.*, 2:863–890.
12. Doniach, I., and Morgan, A. G. (1973): Islet of Langerhans in juvenile diabetes mellitus. *Clin. Endocrinol.*, 2:233–248.
13. Fajans, S. S., Cloutier, M. C., and Crowther, R. L. (1978): The Banting Memorial Lecture 1978, Clinical and etiological heterogeneity of idiopathic diabetes mellitus. *Diabetes*, 27:1112–1125.
14. Fajans, S. S. (1980): Heterogeneity of plasma IRI responses in patients with IGT and diabetes. *Diabetologia*, 19:250.
15. Gepts, W. (1958): Die histopathologischen Veränderungen der Langerhansschen Inseln und ihre Bedeutung in der Frage der Pathogenese des menschlichen Diabetes. *Endokrinologie*, 36:185–211.
16. Gepts, W. (1965): Pathologic anatomy of the pancreas in juvenile diabetes mellitus. *Diabetes*, 14:619–633.
17. Gepts, W., and Toussaint, D. (1967): Spontaneous diabetes in dogs and cats. A pathological study. *Diabetologia*, 3:249–265.
18. Gepts, W., De Mey, J., and Marichal-Pipeleers, M. (1977): Hyperplasia of "Pancreatic Polypeptide"-cells in the pancreas of juvenile diabetics. *Diabetologia*, 13:27–34.
19. Gepts, W., and De Mey, J. (1978): Islet cell survival determined by morphology. An immunocytochemical study of the islets of Langerhans in juvenile diabetes mellitus. *Diabetes, Suppl. 1*, 27:251–261.
20. Gepts, W., and LeCompte, P. (1981): The pancreatic islets in diabetes. *Am. J. Med.*, 70:105–115.
21. Gladisch, R., Bayer, H. P., Lipinski, C., and Stenzel, M. (1975): Insulitis und perakuter Diabetes mellitus. *Z. Kinderheilk.*, 119:5–14.
22. Gorsuch, A. N., Spencer, K. M., Lister, J., McNally, J. M., Dean, B. M., and Botazzo, G. J. (1981): Evidence for a long prediabetic period in type I (insulin-dependent) diabetes mellitus. *Lancet*, 2:1363–1365.
23. Heding, L. G., and Rasmussen, S. M. (1975): C-peptide in normal and diabetic subjects. *Diabetologia*, 11:201–206.
24. Jenson, A. B., Rosenberg, H. S., and Notkins, A. L. (1980): Pancreatic islet cell damage in children with fatal viral infections. *Lancet*, 2:354–358.
25. Junker, K., Egeberg, J., Kromann, H., and Nerup, J. (1977): An autopsy study of the islets of Langerhans in acute-onset juvenile diabetes mellitus. *Acta Path. Microbiol. Scand. (Sect. A)*, 85:699–706.
26. Kawanishi, H., Akazawa, Y., and Machii, B. (1966): Islets of Langerhans in normal and diabetic humans. *Acta Pathol. Jpn.*, 16:177–197.
27. Klöppel, G. (1981): Endokrines Pankreas und Diabetes Mellitus. In: *Spezielle Pathologische Anatomie*. Herausgegeben von W. Doerr und G. Seifert, Band 14, Pathologie der endokrinen Organe, p. 579. Springer Verlag, Berlin, Heidelberg, New York.
28. Kolb, H., Freytag, G., Kiesel, U., and Kolb-Bachofen, V. (1980): Spontaneous autoimmune reactions against pancreatic islets in mouse strains with generalized autoimmune disease. *Diabetologia*, 19:216–221.

29. Kolb, H., Kolb-Bachofen, V., Kiesel, U., and Freytag, G. (1980): Autoimmune reactions against B-cells of pancreatic islets as a consequence of immune dysregulation. *Diabetologia*, 19:291, abstract 222.
30. Lazarus, S. S., and Volk, B. W. (1962): *The Pancreas in Human and Experimental Diabetes*. Grune & Stratton, New York.
31. LeCompte, P. M., and Legg, M. A. (1972): Insulitis (lymphocytic infiltration of pancreatic islets) in late-onset diabetes. *Diabetes*, 21:762–769.
32. LeCompte, P. M., and Gepts, W. (1977): The pathology of juvenile diabetes. In: *The Diabetic Pancreas*, edited by B. Volk and K. Wellman, p. 325. Plenum Press, New York and London.
33. Levine, R. (1977): Introduction. In: *The Diabetic Pancreas*, edited by B. W. Volk and K. F. Wellman, pp. XV–XVIII. Plenum Press, New York and London.
34. Like, A. A., Rossini, A. A., Guberski, D. L., Appel, M. C., and Williams, R. M. (1979): Spontaneous diabetes mellitus: reversal and prevention in the BB/W rat with antiserum to rat lymphocytes. *Science*, 206:1421–1423.
35. Like, A. A., Williams, R. M., Kislaukis, E., and Rossini, A. A. (1981): Neonatal thymectomy prevents spontaneous diabetes in biobreeding/Worcester (BB/w) rat. *Clin. Res.*, 29:542 (abstract).
36. MacCallum, W. G. (1907): Hypertrophy of the islands of Langerhans in diabetes mellitus. *Am. J. Med. Sci.*, 133:432–440.
37. Maclean, N., and Ogilvie, R. F. (1959): Observations on the pancreatic islet tissue of young diabetic subjects. *Diabetes*, 8:83–91.
38. Malaisse-Lagae, F., Stefan, Y., Cox, J., Perrelet, A., and Orci, L. (1979): Identification of a lobe in the adult human pancreas rich in pancreatic polypeptide. *Diabetologia*, 17:361–365.
39. Miller, L. V., Stokes, J. D., and Silipat, C. (1978): Diabetes mellitus and autonomic dysfunction after Vacor rodenticide ingestion. *Diabetes Care*, 1:73–76.
40. Nakhooda, A. F., Like, A. A., Chappel, C. I., Wei, C. N., and Marliss, E. B. (1978): The spontaneously diabetic Wistar rat. *Diabetologia*, 14:199–207.
41. Orci, L., and Unger, R. H. (1975): Functional subdivision of islets of Langerhans and possible role of D cells. *Lancet*, 2:1243–1244.
42. Orci, L., Baetens, D., Rufener, C., Amherdt, M., Ravazzola, M., Studer, P., Malaisse-Lagae, F., and Unger, R. H. (1976): Hypertrophy and hyperplasia of somatostatin containing D-cells in diabetes. *Proc. Nat. Acad. Sci. USA.*, 73:1388–1442.
43. Orci, L., Baetens, D., Ravazzola, M., Stefan, L., and Malaisse-Lagae, F. (1976): Pancreatic polypeptide and glucagon: non-random distribution in pancreatic islets. *Life Sci.*, 19:1811–1816.
44. Orci, L., and Unger, R. H. (1977): Possible roles of the pancreatic D cell in the normal and diabetic states. *Diabetes*, 26:241–244.
45. Orci, L., Malaisse-Lagae, F., Baetens, D., and Perrelet, A. (1978): Pancreatic polypeptide rich regions in human pancreas. *Lancet*, 2:1200–1281.
46. Pauluzzi, L. (1963): Sindrome diabetica post-aftosa nel bovino nel caprino. *Clin. Vet. (Milano)*, 86:113–132.

47. Pedini, B., Avellini, G., Morettini, B., and Comodo, N. (1962): Diabete mellito post-aftoso nei bovini. *Atti Soc. Ital. Sci. Vet.*, 16:443–450.
48. Pittman, W. B., Acton, R. T., Barger, B. O., Bell, D. S., Go, R. C. P., Murphy, C. C., and Roseman, J. (1982): HLA-A_1–B_1 and DR associations in type I diabetes mellitus with onset after age forty. *Diabetes*, 31:122–125.
49. Pont, A., Rubino, J. M., Bishop, D., and Peal, R. (1979): Diabetes mellitus and neuropathy following Vacor ingestion in man. *Arch. Intern. Med.*, 139:185–187.
50. Prosser, P. R., and Karam, J. H. (1978): Diabetes mellitus following rodenticide ingestion in man. *J.A.M.A.*, 239:1148–1150.
51. Rahier, J., Wallon, J., and Gepts, W. (1981): Volume of the pancreatic polypeptide (PP) cell rich lobe in the diabetic pancreas. *Diabetologia*, 21:318–319 (abstract).
51a. Rahier, J., Goebbels, R. M., and Henguin, J. C. (1983): Cellular composition of the human diabetic pancreas. *Diabetologia*, 24:366–371.
52. Reaven, G. M., Bernstein, R., Davis et al. (1976): Non-ketotic diabetes mellitus: Insulin deficiency or insulin resistance. *Am. J. Med.*, 60:80–88.
53. Rosenbloom, A. L. (1982): Letter to the Editor. *Lancet*, 1:285.
54. Rossini, A. A., Williams, R. M., Mordes, J. P., Appel, M. C., and Like, A. A. (1979): Spontaneous diabetes in the gnotobiotic BB/W rat. *Diabetes*, 28:1031–1032.
55. Seifert, G. (1959): Die pathologische Morphologie der Langerhansschen Inseln, besonders biem Diabetes mellitus des Menschen. *Verh. Dtsh. Ges. Pathol.*, 18:50–84.
56. Skyler, J. S., and Cahill, G. F. (1981): Diabetes mellitus: Progress and Directions. In: *Diabetes Mellitus*, edited by J. S. Skyler and G. F. Cahill. Foreword. Yorke Medical Books.
57. Toniolo, A., Onodera, T., Yoon, J. W., and Notkins, A. L. (1980): Induction of diabetes by cumulative environmental insults from viruses and chemicals. *Nature*, 288:383–385.
58. Turner, R. C., Matthews, D. R., Holman, R. R., and Peto, J. (1982): Relative contributions of insulin deficiency and insulin resistance in maturity-onset diabetes. *Lancet*, 1:596–598.
59. Unger, R. H. (1976): Diabetes and the alpha cell. The Banting Memorial Lecture. *Diabetes*, 25:136–151.
60. Volk, B. W., and Wellman, K. F. (1977): *The Diabetic Pancreas*. Plenum Press, New York and London.
61. Volk, B. W., and Wellman, K. F. (1980): Pancreatic pathology of maturity-onset diabetes mellitus. In: *Secondary Diabetes. The Spectrum of the Diabetic Syndromes*, edited by S. Podolski and M. Viswanathan, p. 33. Raven Press, New York.
62. Warren, S., LeCompte, P. M., and Legg, M. A. (1966): *The Pathology of Diabetes Mellitus*, 4th ed, pp. 53–101 and 351–354. Lea & Febiger, Philadelphia.
63. Westermark, P., and Grimelius, L. (1973): The pancreatic islet cells in insular amyloidosis in diabetic and non-diabetic adults. *Acta Pathol. Microbiol. Scand. (Sect. C)*, 81:291–300.

64. Westermark, P., and Wilander, E. (1978): The influence of amyloid deposits on the islet volume in maturity-onset diabetes mellitus. *Diabetologia*, 15:417–421.
65. Yoon, J. W., Austin, M., Onodera, T., and Notkins, A. L. (1979): Virus-induced diabetes mellitus: Isolation from a virus from the pancreas of a child with a diabetic ketoacidosis. *N. Engl. J. Med.*, 300:1173–1179.

The Importance of Islets of Langerhans for Modern Endocrinology, edited by K. Federlin and J. Scholtholt, Raven Press, New York © 1984.

Diabetes and Virus

Horst Müntefering

Department of Pediatric Pathology, Institute of Pathology, Johannes Gutenberg University, 6500 Mainz, Federal Republic of Germany

DIABETES AND VIRUS

Since the turn of the century, there has been discussion as to whether diabetes, particularly type I, might not possibly be caused by infection, at least in part. In spite of this discussion, the number of observed cases of permanent diabetes mellitus following a manifest virus infection has stayed confined to rare observations of isolated cases. More frequently, temporary disturbances in islet function were noted, as were the onset of glycosuria and hyperglycemia, or changes in glucose tolerance.

FINDINGS IN HUMANS

Only a small portion of the viruses able to cause pancreatitis in humans (Table 1) can be regarded on the basis of isolated observations or on epidemiological studies as a potential cause of diabetes. Yet, until now, no direct attack on the islet cells by a virus has been proved. Certainly, Prince et al. (41) reported on a replication of mumps viruses in human pancreas cell cultures with a 1% to 5% proportion of β cells and similarly in 60% to 95% of the pancreas cells. Whether in this case the genotype of the tissue donor played a part or not is an open question. At any rate, the fact remains that patients with manifest mumps pancreatitis do not succumb to chronic diabetes any more often than those with pancreatitis from another cause, i.e., 2% at the most (45).

Other virus infections, such as measles, poliomyelitis, influenza, and cytomegalic inclusion disease have been discussed as

111

TABLE 1. *Viruses able to cause pancreatitis in man and being a potential cause of diabetes*

Virus	Host	Organs Involved	References
Mumps	Human, dog, monkey	Parotis, testicle, ovary, CNS, pancreas, thyroid, eye, ear	Craighead, 1975 (12) Boström, 1968 (3) Prince et al., 1978 (41)
Rubella	Human, monkey	Prenatally: all organs Postnatally: skin, lymph nodes	Forrest et al., 1971 (16) Bunnell an Monif, 1972 (4)
Coxsackie B	Human, mouse	Pancreas, CNS, (mostly inapparent infection) myocardium, pericardium, meningitis	Kibrick and Benirshke, 1958 (28) Yoon et al., 1979 (50) Gladisch et al., 1976 (20) Champsaur et al., 1980 (8)
Foot-and-mouth disease (virus)	Human, cow	Mouth, foot, myocardium, pancreas	Barboni, 1962 (1)
Cytomegalovirus	Human	All organs incl. pancreatic acinar and insular cells	Cappell and McFarlane, 1947 (7)
Infectious mononucleosis	Human	Pancreas	Wislocki, 1966 (48) Everett et al., 1969 (15)
Varicella	Human	Skin, lung, pancreas	Johnson, 1940 (27) Oppenheimer, 1944 (39) Cheatham et al., 1956 (9) Blattner, 1957 (2)

causative factors in isolated cases. The evidence gained from these observations is, however, controversial (3,7).

It is possible that congenital infection with rubella is of greater significance, whereas postnatal infection obviously has no part in the causation of diabetes. Thus, Forrest and Menser (16), following up a collective group of young adults with embryopathia rubeolaris, found that 20% had developed diabetes. This study has since been continued and supplemented by animal experiments.

In 1969, Gamble et al. (18) drew attention to the possible importance of the coxsackie B 4 group of viruses in the development of diabetes. They found clear parallels between the frequency values for juvenile diabetes and the number of coxsackie B 4 infections. In further epidemiological study, Gamble and Taylor (19) showed that the first 3 months after diabetes has become manifest, antibody titers are clearly more often raised. These findings could not be confirmed in several other studies.

Using the case material in Düsseldorf, we also pursued the question of a possible infection with coxsackie B 4 as a causative factor. The decrease in LAH-antibody titer, which is only raised for a short period after infection, would have proved the existence of an infection that had taken its course in the months immediately preceding the onset of manifest diabetes. However, the values listed in Fig. 1 in detail do not indicate any such decrease, so that a coxsackie B 4 infection is not the probable cause of diabetes in those patients examined, until now. Similar frequency values have been found for the coxsackie virus groups B 1, B 2, B 3, and B 5 (44). Yet, there may be a variety of viruses having the ability to damage the B cells of the islets—depending on the genotype, sex, age, and immunological status of the host. However, the problem in discovering the viruses, or that one particular virus, is rooted in the fact that certain subtypes of a virus may be diabetogenic, and these cannot be distinguished from those which are not diabetogenic by the usual diagnostic methods.

We experienced this sort of thing recently with the M-variant of EMC-virus. Using the plaque-purifying method, we found subtypes that caused diabetes in DBA/2 mice, and subtypes which did not. Even in those pools that were subsequently taken

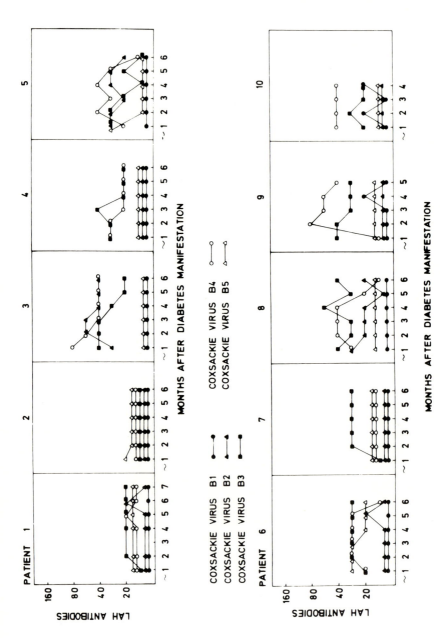

FIG. 1. Course of latex agglutination-inhibiting antibodies from patient with juvenile diabetes.

from diabetic animals, nondiabetogenic subtypes were isolated (see Fig. 6). Thus, epidemiological studies are able to provide a conclusive answer only by positive findings; if, for example, not one single diabetic is found in an epidemic with coxsackie B 4, this does not mean that a subtype of the same virus could not cause diabetes.

So, the only way is to try to isolate a virus from the pancreas of children dying from acute-onset diabetes. In 1979, Yoon et al. (50) obtained material from such a case: a healthy 10-year-old boy was admitted in the hospital in diabetic ketoacidosis within 3 days of the onset of a flu-like illness. Despite intensive therapy, the child's condition deteriorated, and died 7 days later. At autopsy, morphologically, the well-known islet lesion of type I diabetes was observed, with a fulminant course represented by necrosis and infiltrates of macrophages, polymorphs, and lymphocytes within the islets of Langerhans (Fig. 2). The picture

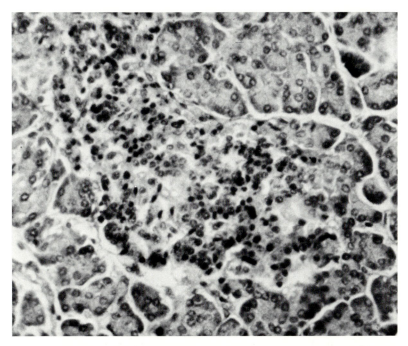

FIG. 2. Islet in the pancreas of a 13-year-old girl with type I diabetes of rapid course and ketoacidosis showing disseminated necroses of islet cells and insulitis (HE; × 310).

was very similar to that seen in the islets of Langerhans from mice that developed diabetes after infection with a virus. Subsequently, a small piece of the child's pancreas was homogenized and then inoculated into a number of different cell lines. Several days later, a cytopathic effect was observed in several of the cultures, and a variant of coxsackie B 4 was successfully isolated. When several inbred strains of mice were inoculated with the human isolate, SJL/J mice developed diabetes, whereas others did not. Moreover, examination of the pancreas from diabetic mice revealed typical lesions (50).

Support for the idea that viruses can trigger some cases of diabetes in humans has lately been strengthened by two additional case reports. The first case was that of a 16-month-old child who came down with a coxsackie B 5 infection and a few days later developed diabetes (8). This virus, which was isolated from the feces, produced abnormal glucose tolerance tests when inoculated into mice. The second case was a 5-year-old girl who had myocarditis and diabetes 2 to 3 weeks after open-heart surgery (20). At necropsy, her islets showed a lymphocytic infiltrate and β-cell necrosis. By immunofluorescence, coxsackie B 4 viruses were found in the serum.

FINDINGS IN ANIMALS

Several viruses belonging to different virus families are known to be able to induce insulitis-deficient diabetes or pathological glucose tolerance in experimental animals (Table 2). The most convincing data to support a viral etiology of diabetes are derived from work with the M-variant of encephalomyocarditis (EMC) virus (6,14,32). The virus develops its diabetogenic effect depending on age and sex (17) and particularly on the genetic factors of the animals determining susceptibility or resistance to diabetes (13,49).

Most suitable for testing are the DBA/2 male mice, 12 weeks of age. In these mice, 72 hr after subcutaneous infection, necrosis of numerous islet cells occurs, followed by inflammatory infiltration with isolated granulocytes, phagocytes, and a few lymphocytes (Fig. 3). Damage to each islet is of varied severity. At times islets can be found in which only isolated cell necrosis and very sparse infiltrates occur (31). Later on there is a shrinking of the islets and very few inflammatory cells are seen. As a rule, from the 30th day after infection on, at the latest from the 40th day on, the islets are small, no longer round, and free of inflammatory infiltration. At this point, there are no β cells, or at best few β cells, in the islets. The remainder has disappeared completely. Finally, in the chronic stage, the shrunken islets consist of only a few β cells (Fig. 4), the number of A cells and D cells seems considerably increased.

Quantitative examinations on the question as to whether or not a true increase in A and D cells occurred, or whether or not these cells have only shifted together because of the islet's shrinking, are not yet complete. Our results until now indicate that the islet tissue structure has merely collapsed and that there is not a real increase of A and D cells.

Islet measurements showed in chronic diabetes at first a rapid, then gradually decreasing shrinkage of the islet by depletion of the β cells completed between about the 30th and 40th day. As the number of β cells decreases, the blood sugar level rises, and this rise does not follow a linear graph: at approximately 10 cells per islet section, the islet has become insufficient (Fig. 5).

SUBTYPES OF VIRUSES

In susceptible syngenic mice, the development of diabetes after infection with the M-variant of EMC virus is not consistent; sometimes only about 10% to 30% of mice developed diabetes, whereas at other times up to 60% developed diabetes. Statistically significant differences were consistently found on repetition of the same experiment and between cages within experimental groups. Moreover, when this virus was passaged in mouse embryo fibroblast cell cultures, the diabetogenic activity of the virus markedly diminished in contrast to when the virus was passaged in mice. These findings suggested that the stock pool of EMC virus was made up of at least two populations of virus: one having a tropism for insulin-producing β cells and being diabetogenic, and the other not having a tropism for β cells and being nondiabetogenic.

Yoon et al. (51) found by using the plaque-purifying method,

TABLE 2. *Viruses being able to induce diabetes or pathological glucose tolerance in animals*[a]

Virus (type)	Species affected	Pathological changes	References
Coxsackie B (RNA)	Mice	Occasional and fine structural alterations of B cells	Robertson, 1954 (43) Burch et al., 1971 (5) Tsui et al., 1972 (46) Harrison et al., 1972 (22)
Foot-and-mouth disease (RNA)	Cattle	Slight damage in both islets and acinar tissue Almost total absence of islets, with infiltration of round cells and some acinar and ductal necroses	Coleman et al., 1973 (10) 1974 (11) Barboni et al., 1962 (1)
Spontaneous (transmissible agent)	Guinea pig	Degranulation of B cells, and cytoplasmatic inclusions with sparing of A and D cells	Munger and Lang, 1973 (34) Lang and Munger, 1976 (29)
Mumps (RNA)	Monkey (*in vitro*)	Establishment of infection in cultured pancreatic B cells	Prince et al., 1978 (41)
Venezuelan equine encephalomyelitis	Mice (C57KSJ) (db/db)	TC-83 strain, B-cell degranulation and changes in subcellular organelles, especially mitochondria	Goldberg et al., 1978 (21)
Rubella (RNA)	Rabbits	B-cell degranulation and changes in subcellular organelles	Menser et al., 1978 (30)

Reovirus type 1 (RNA)	Mice	Mild B-cell damage and insulitis, with infiltration of mononuclear and plasma cells (in addition: polyendocrine disease)	Onodera et al., 1981 (37) 1982 (38)
Encephalomyocarditis, M-variant (RNA)	Mice	Degranulation and coagulation necrosis with subsequent shrinking of B cells and architectural alterations of islets	Boucher and Notkins, 1973 (6) Craighead, 1975 (12) Craighead and McLane, 1968 (14) Hayashi et al., 1974 (23) Müntefering, 1972 (31)
		Degeneration and necrosis of isolated acinar cells or acinar cells adjacent to the islets of Langerhans	Müntefering et al., 1971 (32) Wellmann et al., 1972 (47)

[a]Modified after Rayfield et al., 1978 (ref. 42).

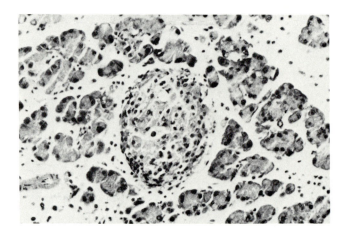

FIG. 3. Section of the pancreas of a 12-week-old mouse 6 days after infection with the M-variant of EMC virus showing disseminated necroses of islet cells and insulitis, but only a mild interstitial pancreatitis (HE; × 200).

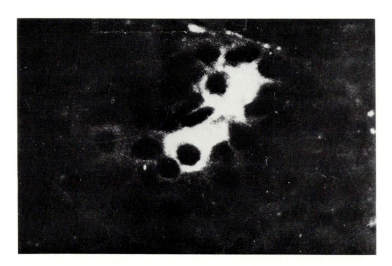

FIG. 4. A shrunk islet in the pancreas of a male DBA/2 mouse in the chronic stage of diabetes 16 weeks after the infection with the M-variant of EMC virus showing only a very few remaining β-cells. (Indirect immunofluorescence; × 500).

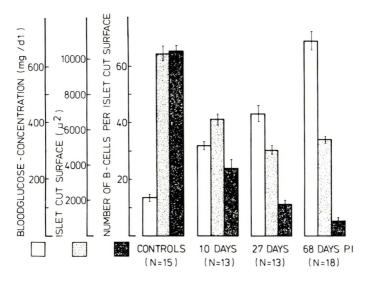

FIG. 5. Blood glucose concentration, size of the islets, and number of β-cells per islets of 15 control animals and of 44 DBA/2 mice, diabetic after infection with EMC virus. (Arithmetical mean and standard error of the mean)

several strains, one, C variant, was nonbeta-cytotropic; another one, D-variant, was highly beta-cytotropic (Fig. 6, top). Standard virological techniques, radioimmunoassay included, failed to reveal any differences between the two variants. Meanwhile, we ourselves have found some more subtypes of the D-variant, many of them being non-beta-cytotropic, like the C-variant of Yoon (Fig. 6, bottom). These findings illustrate the potential difficulty in identifying diabetogenic viruses in nature.

INSULITIS

Inflammation of the islets of Langerhans, or insulitis, as recognized in the juvenile type of diabetes in humans, and also in the EMC-virus-induced diabetes in mice, is one of the factors that suggests the autoimmune hypothesis as an explanation for the pathogenesis of diabetes. We ourselves, having been able to use X-irradiation to prevent virus diabetes, at least in the early stages after infection, thought of an autoimmune process for the first idea (25).

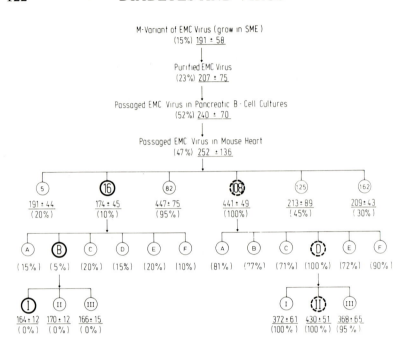

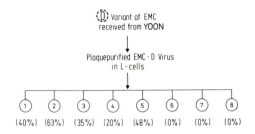

FIG. 6. Top: Isolation of diabetogenic and nondiabetogenic variants EMC virus. The M-variant of EMC virus was passaged five times in murine pancreatic B-cell cultures. The virus then was passaged five additional times in SJL/J male mice. The virus was serially plaque purified. SJL/J male mice were inoculated with virus (5×10^5 PFU) and blood glucose was measured. The mean glucose index of 110 uninfected SJL/J male mice $14^5 \pm 19$ mg/dl. Any mouse with a glucose index greater than 240 mg/dl, which was 5 SD above the mean, was scored diabetic. **Bottom:** Isolation of different subtypes of the D-variant (kindly placed at our disposal by Dr. Yoon). The D-variant was passaged in the same way as described above for the M-variant. ( ), percent diabetic; ———, mean ± SD of glucose index. The data were compiled from 20 mice per group. (From Yoon et al., ref. 51, with permission.)

This opinion was reinforced when we, together with Petersen and his co-workers, were able to prevent virus diabetes by neonatal thymectomy, and we noted that this also prevented the otherwise obligatory insulitis (40). So, we tried to transfer diabetes from infected to normal mice by transfer of lymphocytes. But in our hands, very extensive experiments, in which various modifications of transfer were carried out, have never been successful (Fig. 7). What importance should we in this case attach to insulitis in the pathogenesis of diabetes? In order to be able to answer that question, we made a quantitative analysis of the phenomenon "insulitis." What we found is that the intensity of inflammatory infiltration shows two peaks in the course of infection: one of the early postinfection phase and one during the third week (Fig. 8). But the infiltrates of the two phases are different. In the first week, one finds numerous necrotic and pyknotic cells. During this phase, the inflammatory infiltrate consists of 95% macrophages, 2% granulocytes, and 3% lymphocytes.

Between the 8th and the 22nd day, the necroses have been amply disposed of, and so the phagocytes recede. That result means that afterward, in most animals, no further infiltrates can be observed. The few infiltrates, which are still to be found, consist for the most part of lymphocytes, after the 25th day, to 100%. After the 31st day in this experiment, after the 40th day at the latest in others, there were no infiltrates at all to be found. The intensity of the infiltrates in the second phase is on principle essentially smaller than in the first phase.

We would interpret this phenomenon of the biphasic course as follows: The first phase is obviously to be considered as an unspecific reaction to the lesion caused by the virus and as an unspecific disposal reaction. The second phase could be regarded as a sign of a specific reaction in the context of an immunological process. The number of immune competent cells involved is, as a rule, so small that this factor can only be significant when there is a great deal of preliminary damage to the islet tissue. It must, however, be emphasized that the small intensity and the always transitory nature of the inflammatory infiltrates provide evidence against a classical immunological

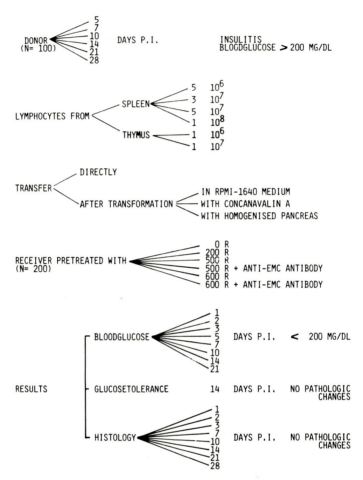

FIG. 7. Transfer of lymphocytes from male DBA/2 mice with virus diabetes. The picture shows a survey of eight different experiments. Lymphocytes from a total of 100 donors were transferred to a total of 200 receivers. Thereby, lymphocytes of spleen and thymus were used. The number of cells, the moment of taking the cells, and the pretreatment of the receiver mice were varied. In two of the experiments, there was interposed an *in vitro* culture of lymphocytes added by mitogenetic factors, respectively, homogenized pancreas. A transfer of diabetes succeeded in none of the experiments.

type IV reaction as a cause of the diabetes. If there is a T-cell-mediated or a macrophage-mediated cytotoxicity involved at all, then it is certainly in the sense that only a few cells, which

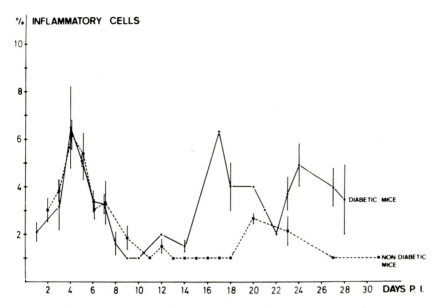

FIG. 8. Number of inflammatory cells per 100 islet cells of at least 100 islets from seven to eight animals each day during the course of the EMC-virus lesion in animals with (———) and without (----) a manifestation of diabetes. Animals that do not develop any diabetes demonstrate insulitis only in the early phase after infection. Only with diabetic animals can one see an infiltration of the islets past the second week.

may remain after the initial damage, are destroyed by them. Thus, in any case a great deal of preliminary damage by the virus itself is necessary.

Therefore, further experiments must clarify whether or not the undoubted significance of the thymus-dependent immune system for the EMC-virus model should not be sought in quite different mechanisms, e.g., an influencing of virus kinetics or other interactions between viruses and the immune system.

Studies of the human pancreas in juvenile-type diabetes have not as yet uncovered any proof of the lymphocytic infiltration well known from other diseases, definitely mediated by T-cells. The insulitis, found in those cases with a rapid course, corresponds in its intensity and cell composition to the insulitis of the EMC-model. For this reason, a classical immunological type IV reaction is not to be expected in humans.

REFERENCES

1. Barboni, E., and Manocchio, I. (1962): Alterazionia pan-pancreatiche in bovini con diabete mellito post-aftoso, *Arch. Vet. Ital.*, 13:477–489.
2. Blattner, R. J. (1957): Serious complications of varicella including fatalities. *J. Pediatr.*, 50:515–517.
3. Boström, K. (1968): Patho-anatomical findings in a case of mumps with pancreatitis, myocarditis, orchitis, epididymitis and seminal vesiculitis. *Virchows Arch.*, 344:111–117.
4. Bunnell, C. E., and Monif, G. R. G. (1972): Interstitial pancreatitis in the congenital rubella syndrome. *J. Pediatr.*, 80:465–466.
5. Burch, G. E., Tsui, C. Y., Harb, J. M., and Colcolough, H. L. (1971): Pathologic findings in the pancreas of mice infected with Coxsackie B 4, *Arch. Intern. Med.*, 128:40–47.
6. Boucher, D. W., and Notkins, A. L. (1973): Virus-induced diabetes mellitus: I. Hyperglycemia and hypoinsulinemia in mice infected with encephalomyocarditis virus, *J. Exp. Med.*, 137:1226–1239.
7. Cappell, D. F., and Mc.Farlane, M. N. (1947): Inclusion bodies (protozoan-like cells) in the organs of infants. *J. Pathol. Bacteriol.*, 59:385–398.
8. Champsaur, H., Dussaix, E., Samolyk, D., Fabre, E., Bach, C. H., and Assan, R. (1980): Diabetes and coxsackie virus B5 infection. *Lancet*, 1:251.
9. Cheatham, W. J., Weller, T. H., Dolan, T. F., and Dower, J. C. (1956): Varicella: report of two fatal cases with necropsy, virus isolation, and serologic studies. *Am. J. Pathol.*, 32:1015–1036.
10. Coleman, T. J., Gamble, D. R., and Taylor, K. W. (1973): Diabetes in mice after coxsackie B4 virus infection, *Br. Med. J.*, 3:25–27.
11. Coleman, T. J., Taylor, K. W., and Gamble, D. R. (1974): The development of diabetes following Coxsackie B virus infection in mice, *Diabetologia*, 10:755–759.
12. Craighead, J. E. (1975): The role of viruses in the pathogenesis of pancreatic disease and diabetes mellitus, *Prog. Med. Virol.*, 19:161–214.
13. Craighead, J. E., and Higgins, D. A. (1974): Genetic influences affecting the occurrence of a diabetes mellitus-like disease in mice infected with the encephalomyocarditis virus, *J. Exp. Med.*, 139:414–426.
14. Craighead, J. E., and McLane, M. F. (1968): Diabetes mellitus: induction in mice by encephalomyocarditis virus, *Science*, 162:913–914.
15. Everett, E. E., Volpe, J. A., and Bergin, J. J. (1969): Pancreatitis in infectious mononucleosis. *South Med. J.*, 62:359–360.
16. Forrest, J. M., Menser, M. A., and Burgess, J. A. (1971): High frequency of diabetes mellitus in young adults with congenital rubella. *Lancet*, 2:332–334.
17. Friedman, S. F., Grota, L. J., and Glasgow, L. A. (1972): Differential susceptibility of male and female mice to encephalomyocarditis virus: effects of castration, adrenalectomy, and the administration of sex hormones. *Infect. Immun.*, 5:637–644.
18. Gamble, D. R., Kinsley, M. L., Fitzgerald, M. G., Bolton, R., and Taylor, K. W. (1969): Viral antibodies in diabetes mellitus. *Br. Med. J.*, 3:627–630.

19. Gamble, D. R., and Taylor, K. W. (1969): Seasonal incidence of diabetes mellitus. *Br. Med. J.*, 3:631–633.
20. Gladisch, R., Hoffman, W., and Waldherr, R. (1976): Myokarditis und Insulitis nach Coxsackie-Virus-Infektion. *Z. Kardiol.*, 65:837–849.
21. Goldberg, S. L., Kochicheril, N. M., Schulman, R., Walker, G. F., and Rayfield, E. J. (1978): Venezuelan encephalitis virus-induced defects in carbohydrate metabolism in genetically diabetic mice. *Diabetes (Suppl. 2)*, 27:477.
22. Harrison, A. K., Bauer, S. P., and Murphy, F. A. (1972): Viral pancreatitis: ultra-structural pathological effects of Coxsackie virus B3 infection in newborn mouse pancreas. *Exp. Mol. Pathol.*, 17:206–219.
23. Hayashi, K., Boucher, D. W., and Notkins, A. L. (1974): Virus-induced diabetes mellitus. II. Relationship between beta cell damage and hyperglycemia in mice infected with encephalomyocarditis virus. *Am. J. Pathol.*, 75:91–102.
24. Jansen, F. K. (1980): The possible relationship between viral infection and autoimmunity. In: *Immunology of Diabetes*, edited by J. Irvine, pp. 243–254. Teviot Scientific Publications Ltd., Edinburgh.
25. Jansen, F. K., Müntefering, H., and Schmidt, W. A. K. (1977): Virus induced diabetes and the immune system. I. Suggestion that appearance of diabetes depends on immune reactions, *Diabetologia*, 13:545–549.
26. Jansen, F. K., Müntefering, H., Thurneyssen, O., and Derocq, J. M. (1979a): Possible interaction between viral infection and autoimmunity in Diabetes. *International Congress Series No. 500*, Diabetes 1979, Proceedings of the 10th Congress of the International Diabetes Federation Vienna, Austria, Sept. 9–14, 1979, edited by W. K. Waldhäusl, pp. 373–378. Excerpta Medica, Amsterdam.
27. Johnson, H. N. (1940): Visceral lesions associated with varicella. *Arch. Pathol.*, 30:292–307.
28. Kibrick, S., and Benirschke, K. (1958): Severe generalized disease (encephalo-hepatomyocarditis) occurring in the newborn period and due to infection with Coxsackie virus, group B. *Pediatrics*, 22:857–875.
29. Lang, C. M., and Munger, B. L. (1976): Diabetes mellitus in the guinea pig, *Diabetes*, 25:434–443.
30. Menser, M. A., Forrest, J. M., and Bransby, R. D. (1978): Rubella infection and diabetes mellitus, *Lancet*, 1:57–60.
31. Müntefering, H. (1972): Zur Pathologie des Diabetes mellitus der weiβen Maus bei der EMC-Virusinfektion. Histologische, elektronenmikroskopische und quantitativ-morphologische Befunde an den Langerhansschen Inseln, *Virchows Arch.*, 356:207–234.
32. Müntefering, H., Schmidt, W. A. K., and Körber, W. (1971): Zur Virusgenese des Diabetes mellitus bei der weiβen Maus. *Dtsch. Med. Wochenschr.*, 96:693–697.
33. Müntefering, H., Schmitz, W., Jansen, F. K., and Petersen, K. G. (1979): The role of transitory insulitis in the pathogenesis of experimental virus-diabetes. *International Congress series No. 500*, Diabetes 1979, Proceedings of the 10th Congress of the International Diabetes Federation. Vienna, Austria, Sept. 9–14, 1979, edited by W. K. Waldhäusl, pp. 395–401. Excerpta Medica, Amsterdam.
34. Munger, B. L., and Lang, C. M. (1973): Spontaneous diabetes mellitus

in guinea pigs: the acute cytopathology of the islets of Langerhans. *Lab. Invest.*, 29:285–302.
35. Notkins, A. L. (1977): Virus-induced diabetes: Brief review. *Arch. Virol.*, 54:1.
36. Onodera, T., Jenson, A. B., Yoon, J. W., and Notkins, A. L. (1978): Virus-induced diabetes mellitus: Reovirus infection of Pancreatic β cells in Mice. *Science*, 201:529–531.
37. Onodera, T., Toniolo, A., Ray, U. R., Jenson, A. B., Knazek, R. A., and Notkins, A. L. (1981): Virus-induced diabetes mellitus. XX. Polyendocrinopathy and autoimmunity. *J. Exp. Med.*, 153:1457–1473.
38. Onodera, T., Ray, U. R., Melez, K. A., Suzuki, H., Toniolo, A., and Notkins, A. L. (1982): Virus-induced diabetes mellitus: autoimmunity and polyendocrine disease prevented by immunosuppression. *Nature*, 297:66–68.
39. Oppenheimer, E. H. (1944): Congenital chickenpox with disseminated visceral lesions. *John Hopkins Hosp. Bull.*, 74:240–249.
40. Petersen, K. G., Müntefering, H., Schmidt, W. A. K., Schlüter, K., Kasemir, H., Treiber, A., Herbst, D., and Kerp, L. (1982): Prevention of EMC virus induced diabetes of mice by neonatal thymectomy. *Diabetologia*, (*in press*).
41. Prince, G. A., Jenson, A. B., Billups, L. C., and Notkins, A. L. (1978): Infection of human pancreatic beta cell cultures with mumps virus. *Nature*, 271:158–161.
42. Rayfield, E. J., and Seto, Y. (1978): Viruses and the pathogenesis of diabetes mellitus. *Diabetes*, 27:1126–1142.
43. Robertson, J. S. (1954): The pancreatic lesion in adult mice infected with a strain of pleurodynia virus. I. Electron microscopical observations. *Aust. J. Exp. Biol. Med. Sci.*, 32:393–409.
44. Schmidt, W. A. K., Brade, L., Müntefering, H., and Klein, M. (1978): Course of coxsackie B antibodies during juvenile diabetes. *Med. Microbiol. Immunol.*, 164:291–298.
45. Shumacker, H. B. (1940): Acute pancreatitis and diabetes. *Ann. Surg.*, 112:177–200.
46. Tsui, C. Y., Burch, G. E., and Harb, J. M. (1972): Pancreatitis in mice infected with Coxsackie B1. *Arch. Pathol.*, 93:379–389.
47. Wellmann, K. F., Amsterdam, D., Brancato, P., and Volk, P. W. (1972): Fince structure of pancreatic islets of mice infected with the M variant of the encephalomyocarditis virus. *Diabetologia*, 8:349–357.
48. Wislocki, L. C. (1966): Acute pancreatitis in infectious mononucleosis. *N. Engl. J. Med.*, 275:322–323.
49. Yoon, J-W., and Notkins, A. L. (1976): Virus-induced diabetes mellitus. VI. Genetically determined host differences in the replication of encephalomyocarditis virus in pancreatic beta cells. *J. Exp. Med.*, 143:1170–1185.
50. Yoon, J-W., Austin, M., Onodera, T., and Notkins, A. L. (1979): Virus-induced diabetes mellitus: Isolation of a virus from the pancreas of a child with diabetic Ketoacidosis. *N. Engl. J. Med.*, 300:1173.
51. Yoon, J-W., McClintock, P. R., Onodera, T., and Notkins, A. L. (1980): Virus induced diabetes mellitus. XVIII. Inhibition by non diabetogenic variant of encephalomyocarditis virus. *J. Exp. Med.*, 150:878–892.

The Importance of Islets of Langerhans for Modern Endocrinology, edited by K. Federlin and J. Scholtholt, Raven Press, New York © 1984.

Treatment of Diabetes Mellitus: Oral Hypoglycemic Agents

Sotirios Raptis

Department of Internal Medicine, Evangelismos Hospital, Athens University, Athens, Greece

The treatment of diabetes with tablets has now been practiced on a large scale for exactly 25 years, and as is today apparent, the results have been successful. As early as 1942, Janbon et al. (25) noted hypoglycemic manifestations after administering carbutamide for the treatment of infections. In 1955, Franke and Fuchs (13) were the first to use this sulfonamide for the treatment of diabetes mellitus, an idea for which they deserve great credit. Research on the mechanism of action of sulfonylureas was started as early as 1944 by Loubatières (31) in Montpellier, and he showed that the presence of the pancreas was essential for their hypoglycemic effect. The idea that human diabetes might be caused by abnormalities in the secretion dynamics of insulin was first suggested at the same time as when sulfonylureas had begun to find acceptance—a coincidence that was certainly not due to chance (43,46).

In all diabetic patients, the fundamental and crucial abnormality is the rigid secretion response of the islet system toward rises in blood sugar (43). The hypothesis that the islet system is refractory to rises in blood sugar but responsive to sulfonylureas would undoubtedly reconcile the clinical features of the disease, in particular those of the human maturity-onset diabetes, with the insulinotropic effect of these substances. There is now no longer any reason to doubt that hypoglycemic drugs (sulfonylureas) act by liberating existing but unutilized insulin reserves, as first postulated by Pfeiffer et al. in 1957 (46).

It is therefore understandable that the principles of oral diabetes therapy are based on our present concepts of the pathogenesis of so-called maturity-onset diabetes (type II). At the beginning of the chain of circumstances involved in its pathogenesis are such conditions as obesity, hyperinsulinism, metabolization of fat rather than carbohydrate, and relative insulin resistance. As the result of a genetically predetermined limitation of individual insulin-synthesis capacity, the chronically overstimulated beta cells of the pancreas sooner or later evince a progressive decline in efficiency, the outcome being relative insulin lack.

In contrast to juvenile diabetes (type I), in which insulin production is totally extinct (and there is hence no place for oral therapy with sulfonylureas), there are still substantial reserves of insulin in patients with clinically manifest maturity-onset diabetes, though in relation to the increased demand for insulin their mobilization is both inadequate and delayed. This state of affairs was termed by Pfeiffer et al. (43) as "insulin secretion rigidity" (Fig. 1).

The objective of treatment is to improve or normalize glucose assimilation by oral treatment. This can be accomplished in several ways:
1. By systematic weight reduction.
2. By stimulating insulin secretion with drugs.
3. By giving drugs to slow down the rise in blood sugar induced by food, or to speed up glucose assimilation, without attempting to modify the abnormalities of insulin secretion, and finally to act on insulin receptors at the periphery.

WEIGHT REDUCTION

The ancient Greeks (Aretaeus, 33 BC) were aware that diabetes was a disease of prosperous citizens, in other words, the obese, and that the disease, or at least the polyuria, disappeared when weight was drastically reduced. In modern Greece, as in other countries, there was a significant decline in consultations for diabetes during World War II (8) (Fig. 2). In every general or consulting practice, and even in specialized centers, approximately 80% of diabetics undergoing treatment are overweight

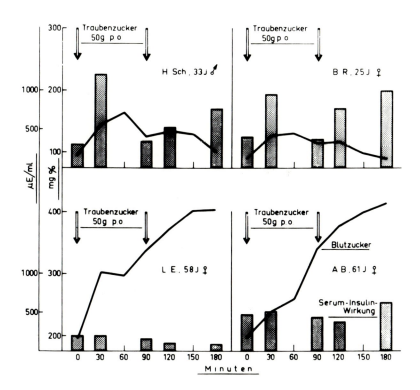

FIG. 1. Blood sugar and insulin-like activity in two normal persons (*upper part*) and in two maturity-onset diabetics (*lower part*). The delay and the rigidity of insulin secretion after glucose administration is characteristic in diabetics. (From Pfeiffer et al., ref. 43, with permission.)

(49). When an obese, maturity-onset diabetic achieves a significant reduction in weight, the blood sugar will often return to normal without any need for further drug treatment. Oral antidiabetics in general and sulfonylureas in particular are therefore unnecessary in a large proportion of this group of obese diabetics.

When these compounds are administered to obese diabetics, their well-known power of stimulating insulin secretion (41,42) leads to transient accentuation of the preexisting hyperinsulinism. This has various consequences, among them, interference

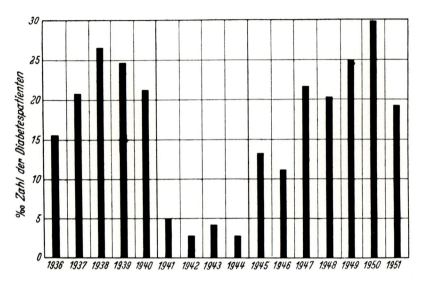

FIG. 2. The number of diabetic patients under treatment in the First Department of Internal Medicine, Athens University, Greece, between the period 1936 to 1951. The decrease of the frequency between the years 1941 to 1944 when there was lack of food during World War II is characteristic. (From Danopoulos and Angelopoulos, ref. 8, with permission.)

with weight reduction. In such patients sulfonylureas can indeed bring the blood sugar down to normal, but other risk factors such as hypertriglyceridemia, hypercholesterolemia, hyperuricemia, and overweight persist and continue to exercise their dire influence on the diabetic's ultimate fate.

In all long-term trials of sulfonylureas and in every attempt to assess the quality of control, the patient's body weight is a factor that must constantly be borne in mind. Follow-up studies over periods exceeding 1 year have recently given evidence that the long-term effect of sulfonylureas can be explained in terms of their extrapancreatic action.

STIMULATION OF INSULIN SECRETION BY DRUGS

Although weight reduction is undoubtedly the most effective and the only logical mode of treatment for the overweight, maturity-onset diabetic, the physician is frequently compelled to compromise, i.e., to prescribe drugs in addition to dietary measures. In everyday practice, especially for the doctor outside the hospital, and to a lesser extent in specialized centers where intensive training of patients can be undertaken, it is extremely difficult and time-consuming to attempt to convince diabetics, most of whom are elderly and have become familiar with their disease over the course of many years, that they must lose weight.

The drugs that stimulate insulin secretion are grouped together under the general heading of "oral antidiabetics." Those nowadays available are: (a) sulfonylurea derivatives, and (b) sulfamidopiridine derivatives (glycodiazine only). These hypoglycemic sulfonamides are listed in Table 1. The new sulfonamide derivatives, all of which belong to the sulfonylurea group, are distinguished by abbreviated chemical designations beginning with the syllable "gli." Another difference from the older drugs is the substantially lower dosage, as shown in Table 2.

In common with other authors, we have demonstrated in numerous investigations that, with the exception of glibenclamide (Euglucon/Daonil), all sulfonamide derivatives act in the same way as tolbutamide (2,7,34,35,38,56,57,58,64). Because of the profusion of sulfonylurea derivatives on the market, the problem is somewhat complicated and it is not easy to say which sulfonylurea is the most effective in the treatment of patients with maturity-onset diabetes. It is our opinion, and indeed the generally accepted view, that maturity-onset diabetes is more

TABLE 1.

Hypoglycemic Sulfonamide Derivatives	
Carbutamide	Nadisan/Invenol
Tolbutamide	Rastinon/Artosin
Glycodiazine	Redul
Chlorpropamide	Diabetoral/Chloronase
Tolazamide	Norglycin
Glibenclamide	Euglucon 5/Daonil
Glibornuride	Glutril/Gluborid
Glisoxepide	Pro-Diaban
Gliquidone	Glurenorm
Glipizide	Glibenese
Gliclazide	Diamicron

TABLE 2.

Maximum Daily Dose	mg
Nadisan/Invenol	1000
Rastinon/Artosin	2000
Redul	1500
Diabetoral/Chloronase	500
Norglycin	1000
Daonil/Euglucon 5	15
Glutril/Gluborid	75
Pro-Diaban	16
Glurenorm	120
Glibenese	15
Diamicron	160

effectively and more physiologically treated with the second-generation sulfonylureas. This expression—the sulfonylureas of the first and second generations—was first used by Pfeiffer in 1970 (40). For reasons that will be readily understood, it has often been misused in the past, and it has nothing to do with the dosage (whether in µg, mg, or g) of the sulfonylureas in question. Second-generation sulfonylureas are those sulfonylureas that differ from tolbutamide in the mode of insulin secretion which they induce or which, when given with glucose, stimulate enhanced insulin liberation and a greater fall in blood sugar. In earlier studies (14,16,50,51,54,56,57,58), carried out *in vivo* and *in vitro*, and in experimental animals and human beings, we conclusively demonstrated that, with the exception of glibenclamide, all sulfonamide derivatives act in the same way as tolbutamide. Irrespectively of blood sugar level, they stimulate the pancreas to produce a single, rapid, and brief discharge of insulin into the blood, which in turn reduces the blood sugar for a short time only (Fig. 3). The secretion of insulin induced by glibenclamide, on the other hand, comes into action more slowly and lasts longer, and therefore produces a considerably deeper and more sustained fall in blood sugar. Not only between glibenclamide and the classical tolbutamide, but between glibenclamide and the newer gliclazide (Fig. 4) exists the same difference. Gliclazide shows the same insulin-secretion pattern as the old tolbutamide of the first generation, whereas glibenclamide

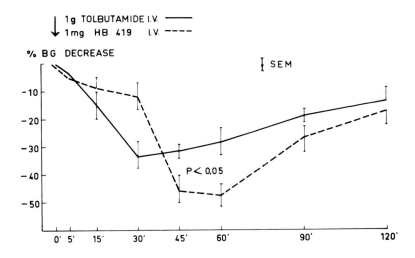

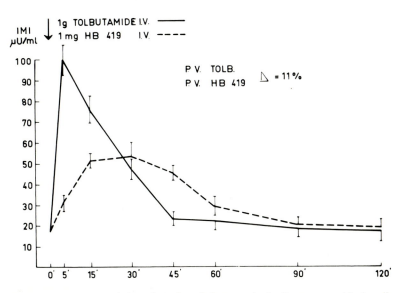

FIG. 3. Blood sugar (*above*) and radioimmunologically measurable insulin (*below*) after administration of tolbutamide or glibenclamide (HB 419). In addition to the steep fall in blood sugar after glibenclamide, note the totally different mode of insulin secretion. (From Raptis et al., ref. 58, with permission.)

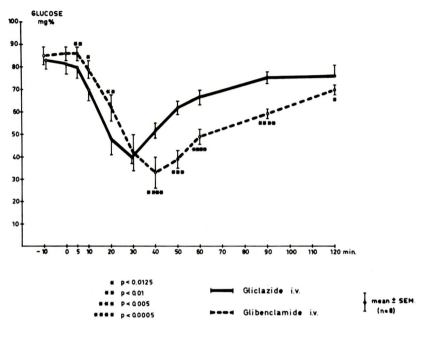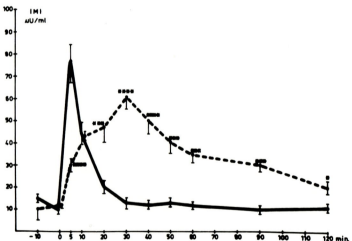

FIG. 4. Blood sugar (*above*) and radioimmunologically measurable insulin (*below*) after administration of gliclazide or glibenclamide (HB 419). In addition to the steep fall in blood sugar after glibenclamide, note the totally different mode of insulin secretion. (From Raptis et al., ref. 58, with permission.)

causes the already described delayed insulin secretion and consequently greater hyperinsulinemia. One special attribute of glibenclamide is that its efficacy is dependent on the blood sugar level, i.e., its insulin-stimulating activity increases in the presence of rising or elevated blood sugar levels, and this is capable of accentuating the rise in insulin induced by food intake, not merely once but indeed repeatedly (Fig. 5). In contrast to that, all sulfonylureas of the first generation with tolbutamide as the main representative are not in a position to cause potentiation of insulin secretion when administered along with glucose (Fig. 6). Opposite to that, after each administration of tolbutamide, a less increase in insulin secretion is caused. In view of this characteristic feature of its action, glibenclamide has been termed the first, and was indeed for a long time the only representative of the second-generation sulfonylureas. All drugs of tolbutamide type are interchangeable with one another. Even in maximum dosage, they are less potent than glibenclamide, which moreover possesses the advantages mentioned above.

It is now generally accepted and is recognized by all investigators in the field that approximately 40% of patients who display secondary failure during conventional oral treatment with first-generation sulfonylureas can be restabilized on glibenclamide. However, this is true of glibenclamide only and does not apply to any other sulfonylurea on the market or undergoing trial (6,19,29,34,50,58,63,68). Furthermore, roughly one-third of maturity-onset diabetics on insulin can be successfully treated with glibenclamide.

When evaluating the data from a large series of diabetics (590 patients) whose illness had first become manifest after the age of 30 years, we found (67) that patients who developed primary or so-called secondary failure on oral therapy were as a rule slender or only slightly overweight (10% above ideal weight). In 38.7% of these patients, it proved possible to continue treatment with glibenclamide, though not with any other sulfonylurea. The most recent work of our research group has shown that up to 43.4% of patients of normal weight developing secondary failure on oral diabetes therapy with sulfonylureas of the first generation (tolbutamide, chlorpropamide, glipizide, and

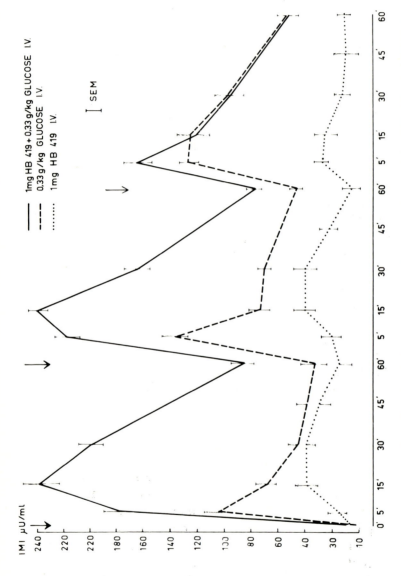

FIG. 5. Insulin secretion after the repeated administration of glucose, glibenclamide (HB 419) and glibenclamide with glucose. The potentiation of the glucose action by the concurrent glibenclamide administration as well as the limited secretion of insulin after the single glibenclamide administration are apparent. (From Raptis et al., ref. 58, with permission.)

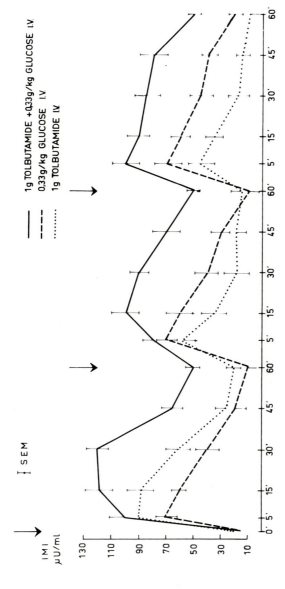

FIG. 6. Insulin secretion after the administration of glucose, tolbutamide and/or combined administration of both. In contrast to glibenclamide (see Fig. 5), tolbutamide is not in a position to cause potentiation of glucose action, not even after repeated administration. Contrary to that, insulin secretion diminishes successively after each tolbutamide administration. (From Raptis et al., ref. 58, with permission.)

gliclazide) can be successfully managed with glibenclamide. Over a period of 24 months, 6.8% of these patients had to be changed over to insulin. Similarly, there were 16 patients with secondary failure on tolbutamide treatment, none of whom achieved restabilization with glipizide (K4024), but continuation of treatment with glibenclamide was successful in 9 of them (Fig. 7). Systematic investigations in which the blood sugar was continuously measured with the aid of the external artificial endocrine pancreas (8,640 measurements in 24 hr) have clearly demonstrated that glibenclamide, in one and the same patient, produces a more physiological blood sugar curve, at least in terms of day and night rhythm, than other sulfonylureas. For example, glibornuride (Fig. 8), gliclazide (Fig. 9), glipizide (Fig. 10), and gliquidone (Fig. 11) produced blood sugar profiles that

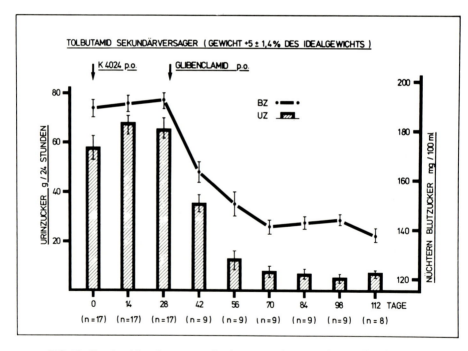

FIG. 7. Fasting blood sugar and urine sugar in 17 patients who developed secondary failure while on tolbutamide treatment and were then changed over to glipizide (K4024). None of the patients was successfully changed over. However, the change over to glibenclamide produced normal blood and urine sugar levels in 9 of the patients.

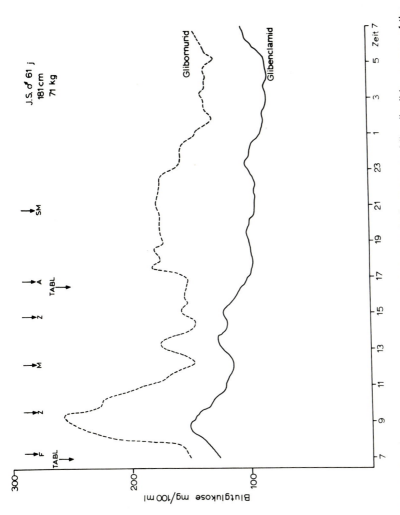

FIG. 8. Continuous blood sugar determinations over 24 hr measured "on line" by means of the artificial endocrine pancreas (Biostator®) in one and the same patient who was treated either with glibenclamide or with glibornuride.

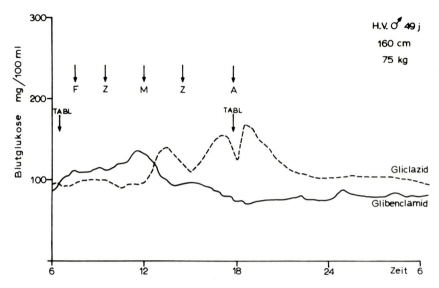

FIG. 9. Continuous blood sugar determinations over 24 hr measured "on line" by means of the artificial endocrine pancreas (Biostator®) in one and the same patient who was treated either with glibenclamide or with gliclazide.

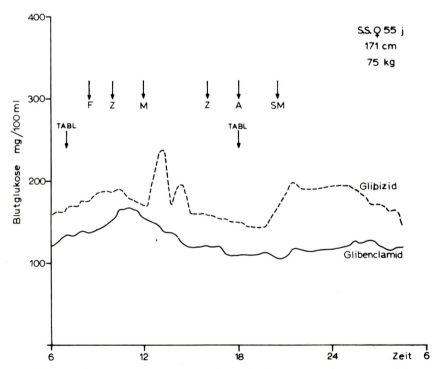

FIG. 10. Continuous blood sugar determination over 24 hr measured "on line" by means of the artificial endocrine pancreas (Biostator®) in one and the same patient who was treated either with glibenclamide or with glipizide.

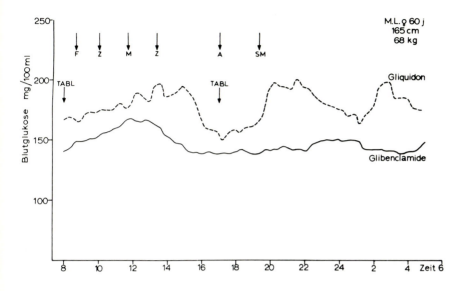

FIG. 11. Continuous blood sugar determinations over 24 hr measured "on line" by means of the artificial endocrine pancreas (Biostator®) in one and the same patient who was treated either with glibenclamide or with gliquidone.

fell far short of those produced by glibenclamide. It goes without saying that these close insights into the behavior of the blood sugar over the 24 hr of the day have become available only since the development of continuous blood sugar measurements. As previously demonstrated (50,52), long-term treatment of maturity-onset diabetics of normal body weight who were given glibenclamide for 6, 9, or 21 months led to an improvement in the blood sugar curve and to some increase in the inadequate rise in insulin secretion (Fig. 12). After treatment was discontinued, glucose tolerance soon became abnormal once again, and it must therefore be assumed that this drug possesses a genuine pharmacological effect, although in humans at least, it does not produce any clinically significant regeneration or new formation of islets.

In the meantime, it has been conclusively demonstrated that maturity-onset diabetics produce an inadequate discharge of insulin in response to a rise in blood sugar. Only in the last few years has it been feasible to obtain objective evidence of this fact, irrespective of whether or not the patient had previously

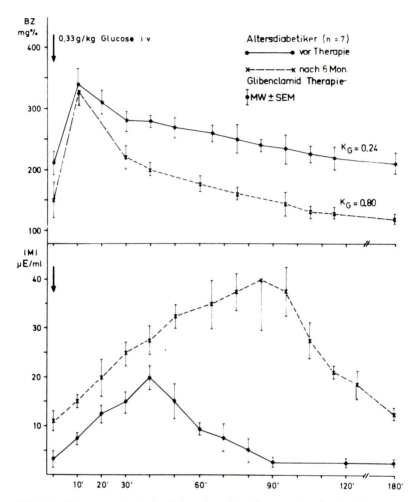

FIG. 12. Glucose assimilation (*above*) and insulin secretion (*below*) in maturity-onset diabetics of normal body weight before and after 6 months glibenclamide treatment. Both the improvement in glucose assimilation and the increase in insulin secretion are clearly recognizable. (From Raptis et al., ref. 61, with permission.)

received insulin and might have insulin antibodies that interfere with the determination of insulin in the blood. The fundamental advance was the discovery of C-peptide, the peptide that links the two chains of the insulin molecule. Measurements of resting values of C-peptide in a large series (235 patients) of maturity-onset diabetics showed that a substantial percentage of these patients still possessed entirely adequate amounts of C-peptide (3). The situation has been made even clearer by maximal stimulation of insulin secretion by combined administration of glibenclamide plus glucose (3,44,45).

By giving combined doses of glibenclamide plus glucose in this way, it is possible to force the pancreas to produce its maximum insulin secretion and indeed to mobilize reserves of insulin that were previously resistant to stimulation by glucose or tolbutamide, alone or in combination (58). This procedure enables us to draw a clear distinction between those diabetics who are still suitable for glibenclamide treatment and those who must have insulin (45,61). If we wish to use this test in a wider clinical context as a means of predicting whether or not the patient will still respond to oral diabetes therapy or whether or not he must be changed over to insulin, it is in fact possible to dispense with insulin assays and to rely solely on the fall in blood sugar (45,61).

If the blood sugar level 3 hr after the combined dose of glibenclamide plus glucose is more than 20% below its initial value (Fig. 13), the change of successful treatment may be estimated at 80%. If we also take into account the absolute and relative insulin values and pick out those patients whose levels have risen more than 500% above the initial insulin value, or if we use the C-peptide level, we can arrive at a successful forecast in almost 90% (4,44,45). This potentiation of a physiological effect, namely, the potentiation of glucose by glibenclamide, has certain consequences during the course of the following day. The insulin level—even after a single dose of the drug given in the morning—will reach its highest values after each meal, and the blood sugar level hence drops to its lowest values at the same times.

This gives 24-hr blood sugar profiles that are quite different from those produced by all other sulfonylureas and are more or less comparable with the blood sugar fluctuations seen in healthy, nondiabetic subjects (7,59,64). Despite this clear mutual adaptation of blood sugar levels and insulin secretion, there is of course no question of any return to the realm of the normal. The

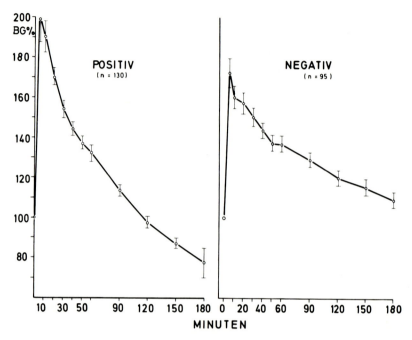

FIG. 13. Blood glucose monitoring for 3 hr after intravenous administration of glibenclamide (1 mg) and glucose (0.33 g/kg BW) in 225 diabetic patients who suffered a secondary failure after sulfonylureas of the first generation. Those patients who had a positive response to the test, i.e., 180 min after the administration of glucose, presented with blood sugar 20% below the starting value (*left*). It was possible to be controlled more satisfactory (80% with glibenclamide). In those who did not show this fall of glucose (*right*), a further treatment with glibenclamide was not possible and they had to receive insulin.

patients are and remain diabetic and any serious dietary indiscretion will be penalized by the expected blood sugar fluctuations. It is not difficult to understand that mobilization of residual insulin from the pancreas by glibenclamide carries with it a danger of hypoglycemia. Nevertheless, practical physicians very swiftly learned how to handle this new and subtle mode of treatment. During the first few years, substantial numbers of hypoglycemic reactions were reported, but in recent years such cases have become less common.

In this context, mention must be made of the interactions between oral antidiabetics and other drugs given at the same time. Interactions may occur with long-acting sulfonamides, barbiturates, salicylates, phenylbutazone, ethionamide, tetracyclines, beta-receptor blockers, reserpine, phenothiazine derivatives, antidepressants, and cumarine derivatives. Special care must be taken in patients with manifest or latent insufficiency of the pituitary-adrenocortical system.

The symptoms and signs of hypoglycemia from oral diabetes treatment vary considerably. In elderly patients the usual manifestations of hypoglycemia such as sweating, sudden hunger, tremor, and paresthesia are often lacking. The picture is dominated by cerebral signs such as confusion, clouding of consciousness, and transient pareses, which may imitate a cerebrovascular accident.

We soon found out that the action of glibenclamide in diabetics does not always become apparent at once (56,57). It often takes 7 to 10 days or even longer to achieve optimal stabilization. It is therefore important not to become discouraged and abandon the drug too soon. When stabilizing a diabetic on glibenclamide, it is absolutely essential to begin with a low initial dose; this can then be gradually raised until the optimum dose is reached. Even in those early days, we noticed that as the treatment was going on, it was necessary to reduce the glibenclamide dose after some time in order to avoid hypoglycemic attacks. It has been postulated that this sulfonylurea has the effect of raising the sensitivity of the beta cells, with the result that they react to smaller rises in blood sugar by secreting greater amounts of insulin (40,50).

A few years later, certain researchers (10,12,), studying overweight, maturity-onset diabetics with pronounced hyperinsulinemia and peripheral insulin resistance, noted that after long-term treatment there was some improvement in glucose tolerance and some breakdown of peripheral insulin resistance. There was no change in body weight during the period of observation.

EXTRAPANCREATIC ACTIONS

From what has just been said, we may reasonably conclude that during long-term administration of glibenclamide to diabetics of normal weight it is in general the pancreatic action of this sulfonylurea that predominates. Over 24 hr the postprandial rise in blood sugar is smoothed out by adequate liberation of insulin (39,54,56,57,64). In obese diabetics the state of affairs is otherwise. In such patients glibenclamide has an extrapancreatic action in addition to its effect on the pancreas. Recent investigations have clearly shown that glibenclamide acts directly on insulin receptors (48). Not only is the affinity of the receptors for insulin enhanced, but there is also a definite increase in the number of insulin receptors per cell, accompanied by normalization of the binding capacity of the peripheral tissues for this hormone. As a result, the derangement of glucose tolerance is compensated and less intrinsic insulin is consumed. These findings also help to explain a fact noted by us 10 years ago, namely, that after some time has elapsed, it is necessary to cut down on the dose of glibenclamide in order to prevent hypoglycemic attacks (50).

Apart from this action of glibenclamide on insulin receptors, we have also shown that it must have an effect on the enteropancreatic axis, this being to some extent independent of its direct pancreatic action. For example, Raptis et al. (55) carried out measurements in portal vein blood after oral administration of glibenclamide to humans and found a rise in insulin and C-peptide before there had been any increase in blood sugar at all. As all known gastrointestinal hormones remained unaffected at this time, we conclude that an unknown gastrointestinal factor was responsible for this early rise in insulin.

These newly discovered extrapancreatic actions of glibenclamide, coming at a time when biguanides have fallen into disfavor and phenformin and buformin have been banned in Germany, can certainly be used for the benefit of patients. So, to demonstrate the clinical value of the extrapancreatic actions of glibenclamide, we gave the drug in small doses to 14 obese diabetics weighing 20% to 30% in excess of normal (Fig. 14). Previously an attempt had been made to treat these patients with diet alone for 3 months (25 cal/kg body weight). As might be expected, they had not lost weight significantly. During the next 3 months the same diet was continued, and they were given 1.25 mg glibenclamide three times daily. Continuous blood sugar recordings over 24-hr periods were made with the artificial pancreas before starting the diet at the end of the period on diet alone and at the end of the glibenclamide period. While the patients were connected to the artificial pancreas, radioimmunological insulin assays were carried out every hour. Glycosylated hemoglobin was also measured at the beginning and end of the diet and glibenclamide periods.

This result yielded clear evidence that glibenclamide, as compared with diet alone, improved the blood sugar curve and diminished hyperinsulinemia (see Fig. 14). No episodes of hypoglycemia were observed in any of the patients. Their body weights remained unaltered. On the basis of these results, it seems reasonable to recommend treatment with small doses of glibenclamide for obese, maturity-onset diabetics who, as is often the case, fail to reduce their weight substantially and whose blood sugar cannot be adequately stabilized by dieting alone.

In view of the positive action of glibenclamide on insulin receptors, it must seriously be considered whether glibenclamide should be given as a supplement to patients displaying insulin resistance or indeed to every patient receiving insulin. Groop and Harfno (18) have in fact shown that administration of sulfonylureas to insulin-dependent diabetics on insulin treatment produces better control of blood sugar. Even more recently (Kerner and Pfeiffer 1981, *unpublished*), systematic investigations with the artificial pancreas have demonstrated that supplementary doses of glibenclamide reduce the insulin requirements of insulin-dependent diabetics. Even in type II diabetes, Bachmann et al. (1) found that combined treatment with insulin and glibenclamide enabled the dose of insulin to be reduced while providing just as good control of blood sugar as insulin alone.

This work naturally prompts the question whether or not any particular diabetic patient would be better treated with insulin or with sulfonylureas. In an attempt to answer this question, we determined the curves of blood sugar and radioimmunologically measurable insulin at 10-min intervals over 24 hr in patients who had been stabilized on insulin (Fig. 15) and who had adequate

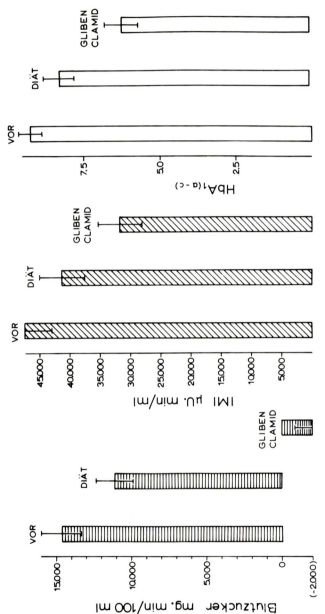

FIG. 14. Blood sugar areas—blood sugar continuously measured "on line" over 24 hr with the artificial endocrine pancreas (Biostator®)—together with radioimmunologically measurable insulin (IMI) and glycosylated hemoglobin (HbA1) in 14 overweight, maturity-onset diabetics who had been treated for 3 months with diet and subsequently for 3 months with the lowest possible doses of glibenclamide. Although the insulin level fell during glibenclamide treatment, there was a considerable improvement in blood sugar and the HbA1 level reverted to normal.

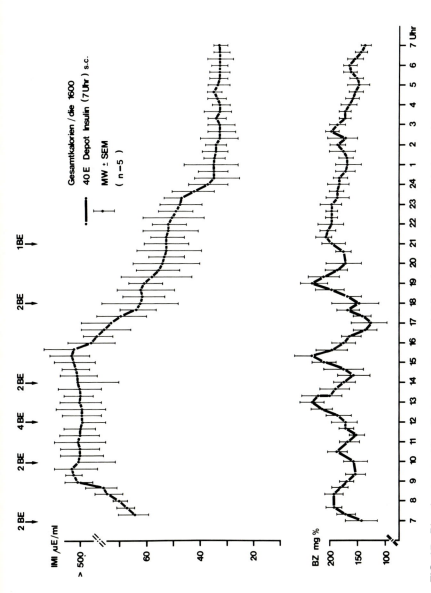

FIG. 15. Blood sugar and insulin curves measured at 10-min intervals over 24 hr in patients who were receiving insulin injections despite that they had still a satisfactory amount of endogenous insulin in their pancreas. (From Raptis et al., ref. 61, with permission.)

intrinsic insulin reserves. They were then treated with glibenclamide (Fig. 16). This produced clear evidence that the fluctuations in blood sugar over 24 hr were smaller during treatment with the oral antidiabetic than they were during treatment with insulin (54). It is therefore advisable, as must be emphasized yet again, that patients who possess adequate insulin reserves and who can be satisfactorily stabilized should on no account be changed over to insulin. Apart from serious renal failure, there is no complication of diabetes that, in the light of our present knowledge, constitutes a sufficient reason for changing a well-stabilized diabetic from sulfonylureas to insulin.

ORAL ANTIDIABETICS AND VASCULAR COMPLICATIONS

A few years ago, it was justifiable to ask, "Do diabetics derive any benefit at all from oral diabetes therapy or do these drugs cause more harm than good?" This apparent dilemma, affecting both doctors and patients, was brought into prominence by an American study group (University Group Diabetes Program—UGDP Study) and in particular by the assertion that oral antidiabetics promote arteriosclerosis (see References for specific works on this topic). This suspicion has proved to be unfounded. Numerous retrospective and prospective trials have failed to confirm these findings and have indeed clearly demonstrated that tolbutamide, for example, postpones the appearance of latent diabetes. Furthermore, not only is angina pectoris less common among diabetics who had been treated with tolbutamide, but also intermittent claudication, myocardial infarcts, and signs of ischemia in the electrocardiogram (20,27,32,37). However, it must always be borne in mind that diabetes mellitus is such an intricate disease and has so many complications, especially in the vascular system, that it is very difficult to disentangle the lesions arising in the natural course of the disease from those that have been produced by medication. A glance at the statistics of the World Health Organization shows amazing variations in mortality among diabetics in different countries throughout the world. There can be no doubt that the length of the protodiabetic stage in maturity-onset diabetics is a

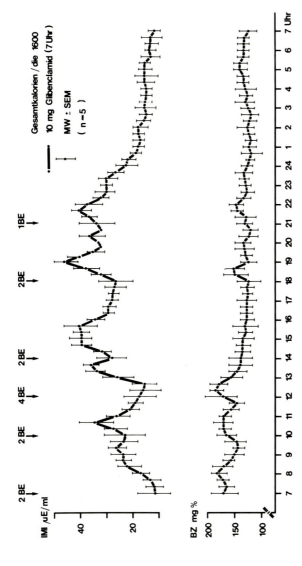

FIG. 16. Blood sugar and insulin curves measured at 10-min intervals over 24 hr in patients (the same as in Fig. 15) who had been changed over from insulin to glibenclamide. The flattening of the fluctuations in blood sugar and the stimulation of insulin secretion after each meal during the period of glibenclamide treatment are clearly recognizable. (From Raptis et al., ref. 61, with permission.)

factor of great importance, especially in regard to the appearance of cardiovascular complications.

Our studies in experimental animals have yielded clear evidence that long-term treatment (up to 1 year) with large doses of various sulfonylureas produces no biochemical or histological abnormalities that arouse the least suspicion that they might promote arteriosclerosis (26). Indeed, Reddi et al. (62), working with rats, demonstrated that long-timed treatment with glibenclamide not only prevented the progression of diabetic glomerulosclerosis, but also led to a significant decrease in glucosyltransferase, the enzyme that in KK-rats is responsible for the development of the genetically predetermined diabetic glomerulosclerosis. More recently, in a study of a large series of diabetics (9), we have demonstrated that beta-thromboglobulin, erythrocyte deformability, and glycosylated hemoglobin display abnormalities that improve when the diabetic state is well controlled—this improvement being irrespective of the mode of therapy.

In the last few years, much effort has been devoted to explaining the beneficial effect of sulfonylureas on the diabetic state and in particular its late complications in terms of their effect on platelet function. Previous personal observations (Raptis, Rasche, Pfeiffer 1976, *unpublished*) leave no doubt that the effects on platelet aggregation observed *in vitro* are of no significance *in vivo*, even over periods of treatment with glyclazide or glibenclamide of more than 16 months' duration. In contrast to these findings, Ponari et al. (47) detected a significant decrease in platelet aggregation after only 3 months of glicaride medication. However, their study had no control group. The clinical relevance of this effect is doubtful. For example, patients with diabetic retinopathy treated by us with gliclazide for 12 months showed no hint of any better response than the control group who received another sulfonylurea and had comparable blood sugar levels. Every ophthalmological follow-up was checked by fluorescence angiography and fundal photography. There is of course no doubt that *in vitro* (28) both gliclazide and glibenclamide and possibly other sulfonylureas have an effect on platelet aggregation, but unfortunately this effect—so far as it is detectable by the current techniques for assessing hemorrheological parameters—remains confined to the *in vitro* "scene."

Lastly, it should perhaps be mentioned that the thyrostatic action of sulfonylureas postulated a few years ago has proved to be illusory. Long-term trials in human patients and experimental animals alike failed to show any abnormality in the secretion of thyroid hormones, and the integrity of the pituitary-thyroid axis has been proved by the TRH test (54).

BIGUANIDES AND ACARBOSE

The incidence of side effects from biguanides is considerably higher than from sulfonylureas. The commonest side effects are loss of appetite, nausea, metallic taste, and diarrhea. The high incidence of lactic acidosis among patients receiving biguanides was the subject of active debate 3 years ago (5, 33), but it is by no means a new discovery, having been known since the introduction of this mode of treatment (69). In our opinion, provided these drugs are used correctly, the risk of lactic acidosis is negligible. It may also be said that a suspicion voiced during the UGDP trial, namely, that biguanides, like sulfonylureas, favor the development of arteriosclerosis, has now been refuted (15, 27, 72).

There are of course certain absolute contraindications—primarily renal, hepatic, or cardiac failure—but provided they are duly observed, biguanides are valuable drugs, especially for overweight, maturity-onset diabetics, and can be used either alone or in combination with sulfonylureas. It is well known that biguanides have an extrapancreatic action. The exact mechanism of action of this group of drugs has not yet been fully clarified. They inhibit lipogenesis, restrict gluconeogenesis, interfere with carbohydrate absorption, and reduce appetite. All these effects are now thought to be responsible for the improvement in carbohydrate metabolism. Recent investigations have also been shown that biguanides are capable of increasing the number of insulin receptors on human erythrocytes (24).

It has been claimed that metformin causes less lactic acidosis than phenformin and buformin, but this may be due to a simple arithmetical error, no account having been taken of the fact that there are far fewer patients receiving metformin than phenformin (ratio approximately 2 to 10). It can therefore be concluded that the same limitations apply to all three biguanides. The banning of biguanides in certain countries is not an irreplaceable loss because first, it has now been proved that glibenclamide in small doses is as good as or even better than biguanides in obese diabetics, and second, because drugs such as acarbose have been developed that delay the absorption of carbohydrates from the gut.

Acarbose is a new glycoside hydrolase inhibitor with special inhibitory activity against sucrose. *In vivo*, acarbose also inhibits the intestinal breakdown of starch and dextrins (22,66). In nondiabetic subjects, acarbose significantly inhibits the rise of blood sugar, insulin, and triglycerides (23). Given in conjunction with oral antidiabetics, acarbose leads to better stabilization in diabetic patients (65). In insulin-dependent diabetics (53), supplementary treatment with acarbose flattens the peaks in the blood sugar curve, as measured by means of the artificial endocrine pancreas, and considerably reduces the daily dose of insulin required.

In view of what has been said above, we consider that there is no reason to modify the list of indications for oral antidiabetics. The sequence of modes of therapy remains unaltered, i.e., first treatment with diet, then diet and tablets, and finally diet and insulin. It may be emphasized yet again as a principle of oral diabetes therapy that weight reduction alone will effect a substantial improvement in the metabolic state of nearly every overweight, maturity-onset diabetic patient. Every doctor in clinical practice should be familiar with this step-by-step plan. Thanks to our new knowledge of the effect of glibenclamide on insulin receptors, this drug can now be used even in overweight patients, provided the dose is adjusted to individual requirements. The use of drugs that delay absorption of carbohydrates from the intestine can also make a substantial contribution to the ideal stabilization of the diabetic patient. However, it must be borne in mind that mere normalization of blood sugar is not the only yardstick for assessing the merits of ideal diabetes therapy. Fat metabolism and reduction of body weight toward normal must also be taken into account. Physicians who do not pay proper attention to all three criteria lay themselves open to the reproach that they are merely treating the blood sugar curve and ignoring the wider aspects of the disease. Under such conditions, arteriosclerosis will progress and the patient will be at risk of cardiovascular complications, as was noted in the American trial among those patients who were treated with diet alone. It may well be true that, after an attempt at dietary treatment has miscarried, only the subsequent correct administration of oral antidiabetics for very long periods will be of value. In regard to the inevitable late complications of diabetes, we cannot afford to neglect any measure that will achieve smoother control of blood sugar levels and hence help to postpone the onset of vascular and neurological complications.

SUMMARY

In contrast to biguanides, sulfonylureas stimulate insulin secretion and break down the rigid insulin-secretion pattern of the maturity-onset diabetic. Sulfonylureas also act on insulin receptors. For this reason, they reduce insulin requirements and can therefore be used even in overweight diabetics. The main emphasis in oral diabetes therapy is centered on the sulfonylurea of the second-generation glibenclamide. Substances that delay the absorption of carbohydrates from the small intestine are used as adjuvants in oral diabetes treatment.

There can be no doubt that there will be a place for oral antidiabetics in the foreseeable future.

ACKNOWLEDGMENTS

The original investigations on which this study is based were carried out with support from the Social Ministry, Athens, Greece; the German Research Association (SFB 87-Endokrinologie-Ulm), Bonn-Bad Godesberg; and the Alexander S. Onassis Foundation, Vaduz-Liechtenstein.

REFERENCES

1. Bachmann, W., Sieger, C., Haslbeck, M., and Lotz, N. (1981): Combination of insulin and glibenclamide (gl) in the treatment of adult-onset diabetes (Type 2). *Diabetologia*, 21:245.
2. Bauer, G., and Kloppe, W. (1969): Ein Beitrag zur Ersteinstellung diätetisch erfolglos vorbehandelter Diabetiker au Englucon 5 (HB 419) (A contribution to the primary stabilization of diabetics on Euglucon 5 (HB 419) after unsuccessful attempts at dietary treatment). *Dtsch. Med. J.*, 20:584–585.
3. Beischer, W., Kerner, W., Raptis, S., Keller, L., Beischer, B., and Pfeiffer, E. F.: Insulin therapy in relation to circulating C-peptide levels. *Diabetes*, 27:235–240.
4. Beischer, W., Raptis, S., Keller, L., Maas, M., Beischer, B., Feilen, K., and Pfeiffer, E. F. (1978): Humanes C-Peptid. Teil III: Sekretionsdynamik der Beta-Zellen erwachsener Diabetikernach Glibenclamid-Glucose i.v. (Human C-peptides. Part III: Secretion dynamics of the beta-cells of maturity-onset diabetics after glibenclamide and glucose i.v.). *Klin. Wochenschr.*, 56:111–120.
5. Berger, W., and Amrein, R. (1978): Laktatazidosen unter der Behandlung mit den drei Biguanidpräparaten Phenformin, Buformin und Metformin-Resultate einer gesamtschweizerischen Umfrage 1977 (Lactic acidoses during treatment with the three biguanides phenformin, buformin and metformin. The results of a questionnaire covering the whole of Switzerland). *Schweiz. Rundschau. Med. (Praxis)*, 67:661–679.
6. Beyer, J., Ewald, W., Kunkel, W., Wolf, E., and Schöffling, K. (1971): Fortschritte der Diabetes-Therapie durch Behandlung mit Glibenclamid und Phenformin (Progress in diabetes therapy by treatment with glibenclamide and phenformin). *Dtsch. Med. Wochenschr.* 96:728–733.
7. Chandalia, H. B., Hollobaugh, S. L., Pennington, L. F., and Boshell, B. R. (1969): Use of glibenclamide in maturity-onset diabetes. Effect of the drug on serum insulin levels. *Horm. Metab. Res. (Suppl.)*, 1:73–76.
8. Danopoulos, E., and Angelopoulos, B. (1953): Vergleichende Untersuchungen über die veränderung des diabetes in den Vorkriegs-, Kriegs- und nachkriegsjahren in Griechenland (Comparative investigations of the changes in diabetes in Greece in the years before, during and after the war.) *Klin. Wochenschr.*, 31:1076–1077.
9. Diamantopoulos, E. J., Raptis, S., Mandel, R., Karaiskos, K., and Moulopoulos, S. (1981): Das Verhalten von β-Thromboglobulin (β-TG), Erythrozyten deformabilität (ED) und glykosiliertem Hämoglobin (GHbA$_1$) bei Diabetikern unter verschiedener Therapieform (The behavior of beta-thromboglobulin (β-TG), erythrocyte deformability (ED), and glycosilated hemoglobin (GHbA$_1$) in diabetics receiving various forms of therapy). *Akt. Endokrinol. Stoff.*, 2:87.
10. Ebert, R., Frerichs, H., and Creutzfeldt, W. (1976): Der Einfluss von Glibenclamid auf die Serumspiegel von gastric inhibitory polypeptide "GIP" und Insulin bei Gesunden und Alters-diabetikern (The influence of glibenclamide on the serum level of "gastric inhibitory polypeptide" [GIP] and insulin in healthy subjects and maturity-onset diabetics). *Dtsch. Diab. Ges.*, 11. Kongr., Braunlage, 1976 Kongressbericht Vortrag No. 10.

11. Efendic, S., Enzmann, F., and Luft, R. (1978): Glibenclamide enhances glucose and arginine stimulated somatostatin release and suppresses the effect of arginine on glucagon release from perfused rat pancreas. *Diabetes*, 28:403.
12. Feldman, J. M., Lebovitz, F. L. (1975): Effect of prolonged administration of glyburide on insulin secretion and glucose tolerance of patients with diabetes mellitus. In: *Micronase (glyburide) pharmacological and clinical evaluation*, edited by H. Rifkin, Excerpta Medica ICS 382:64–76. Amsterdam.
13. Franke, H., and Fuchs, J. (1955): Ein neues antidiabetisches Prinzip (A new antidiabetic principle). *Dtsch. Med. Wochenschr.*, 80:1449–1454.
14. Fussgänger, R. D., Goberna, R., Hinz, M., Jaros, P., Karsten, C., Pfeiffer, E. F., and Raptis, S. (1969): Comparative studies on the dynamics of insulin secretion following HB 419 and tolbutamide of the perfused isolated rat pancreas and the perfused isolated pieces and islets of rat pancreas. *Horm. Metab. Res. (Suppl.)*, 1:34–40.
15. Gilbert, J. P., Saracci, R., Meier, P., Zelen, M., Rümke, C., and White, C. (1975): Report of the Committee for the Assessment of Biometric Aspects of Controlled Trials of Hypoglycemic Agents. *J.A.M.A.* 231:583–608.
16. Goberna, R., Fussgänger, R. D., Raptis, S., Ditschuneit, H., and Pfeiffer, E. F. (1969): Glybenclamide (HB 419) and the prediabetes of subtotally pancreatectomized rats. *Horm. Metab. Res.*, 1:175–177.
17. Gottesbüren, H., Gerdes, H., and Littmann, K.P. (1970): Schwere Hypoglykämien nach Glibenclamid (Severe hypoglycaemic attacks after glibenclamide). 76. Kongress Deutsch. *Ges. Inn. Med.*, 433–435.
18. Groop, L., and Harno, K.: The combination of insulin and sulfonylureas—an approach to improved metabolic control in insulin resistant diabetics. *Acta Endocrinol., (Suppl.)* 91:227.
19. Gutsche, H. (1972): Orale Diabetestherapie (Oral diabetes therapy) *Dtsch. Med. J.*, 23:449–452.
20. Haller, H., and Strauzenberg, S. E. (1967): Sulfonylharnstoffbehandlung des Diabetes mellitus, Spätergebnisse nach 12 Jahren (Sulphonylurea treatment of diabetes mellitus. Late results after 12 years). *Ber. Ges. Inn. Med.*, 5:215.
21. Henning, B. N., Pedersen, O., and Lindskov, H. O. (1979): Increased insulin sensitivity and cellular insulin binding in obese diabetics following treatment with glibenclamide. *Acta Endocrinol.*, 90:451–462.
22. Hillebrand, I., Boehme, K., Frank, G., Fink, H., and Berchtold, P. (1978): Effects of the glucoside-hydrolase inhibitor BAY-g-5421 on postprandial blood glucose, serum insulin, and triglyceride levels: dose-time relationships in man. *Diabetologia*, 15:239–243.
23. Hillebrand, I., Boehme, K., Frank, G., Fink, H., and Berchtold, P. (1979): The effects of the α-glucosidase Inhibitor BAY-g-5421 (Acarbose) on postprandial blood glucose, serum insulin and triglyceride levels: dose-time-response relationships in man. *Res. Exp. Med. (Berl.)*, 175:87–94.
24. Holle, A., Mangels, W., Dreyer, M., Kühnau, J., and Rüdiger, H. W. (1981): Biguanide treatment increases the number of insulin-receptor sites on human erythrocytes. *N. Engl. J. Med.*, 305:563–566.

25. Janbon, M., Chaptal, J., Vedel, A., and Schaap, J. (1942): Accidents hypoglycémiques graves par un sulfamino-thiodiazol (le V.K. 57 ou 2254 R.P.) [Serious hypoglycaemic attacks caused by a sulfaminothiodiazol (V.K. 57 or 2254 R.P.)]. *Soc. Sci. Méd. Biol.* (Montpellier) 222:441.
26. Kamenisch, W., Laube, H., Raptis, S., Mohr, W., and Faulhaber, J. D. (1975): Biochemische und histologische Untersuchungen über die Langzeitwirkung von Sulfonylharnstoffen bei Ratten (Biochemical and histological studies of the long-term effect of sulphonylureas in rats). 10. Kongr Deutsch. Diab. Gesellschaft Ulm, *Nov. Inf. Vortrag,* Nr. 36.
27. Kilo, C., Miller, Ph., and Williamson, J. R. (1980): The achilles heel of the university group diabetes program. *J.A.M.A.* 243:450–457.
28. Klaff, L. J., Kernoff, L., Vinik, A. I., Jackson, W. P. U., and Jacobs, P. (1981): Sulfonylureas and platelet function. *Am. J. Med.,* 70:627–636.
29. Knick, B., Wendt, O., Konder, M. L., and Netter, P. (1970): Orale antidiabetische Mono- und Kombinationstherapie mit Glibenclamid-HB 419 und Biguaniden bei insulinierten Diabetikern des Erwachsenentyps (Oral antidiabetic monotherapy and combined therapy with glibenclamide (HB 419) and biguanides in insulin-treated diabetics of maturity-onset type) *Med. Klin.* 65:109–112.
30. Królewski, A. S., Czyzyk, D., Janeczko, D., and Kopczyński (1977): Mortality from Cardiovascular Diseases among Diabetics. *Diabetologia,* 13:345–350.
31. Loubatières, A. (1944): Relations de mécanisme de l'action hypoglycémiante du p-aminobenzene-sulfamido-isopropyl-thiodiazol (2254 RP) (Relations of the mechanism of hypoglycaemic action of p-aminobenzene-sulfamido-isopropyl-thiodiazol (2254 RP)) *Compt. Rend. Soc. Biol.,* 138:766–773.
32. Lozano-Castaneda, D.: Tolbutamide after 10 years. Brook Lodge Conference, Kalamazoo, Michigan, March 6–7, 1967. Excerpta Medica ICS 149:298–307.
33. Luft, D., Schmülling, R. M., and Eggstein, M. (1978): Lactic acidosis in biguanide-treated diabetics. A review of 330 cases. *Diabetologia,* 14:75–83.
34. Mehnert, H., and Karg, E.: Glybenclamid (HB419) (1969): ein neues orales Antidiabetikum der Sulfonylharnstoff-Reihe (Glibenclamide (HB 419): a new oral antidiabetic of the sulphonylurea series). *Dtsch. Med. Wochenschr.,* 94:819–824.
35. Müller, R., Bauer, G., Schröder, R., and Saito, S. (1969): Summary report of clinical investigation of the oral antidiabetic drug HB 419 (glibenclamide). *Horm. Metab. Res. (Suppl.)* 1:88–92.
36. Owens, D. R., Biggs, P. I., Shetty, K. J., and Wragg, K. G. (1980): The effect of Glibenclamide on the glucose and insulin profile in maturity-onset diabetics following both acute and long term treatment. *Diabetes Metab.,* 6:219–224.
37. Paasikivi, J. (1970): Long-term tolbutamide treatment after myocardial infarction. A clinical and biochemical study of 178 patients without overt diabetes. *Acta Med. Scand. (Suppl.),* 507.
38. Pfeiffer, E. F. (1971): Fortschritte der Diabetologie (Advances in diabetology). *Therapiewoche,* 21:553–561.

39. Pfeiffer, E. F. (1979): Möglichkeiten und Grenzen der medikamentösen Diabetestherapie (Potentialities and limitations of the drug treatment of diabetes). *Therapiewoche*, 29:8310–8321.
40. Pfeiffer, E. F. (1970): Diabetes-Therapie (Diabetes therapy). *Münch. Med. Wochenschr.*, 40:1835–1836.
41. Pfeiffer, E. F., Ditschuneit, H., and Schöffling, K. (1959): Über die bestimmung von Insulin im Blut am epididymalen Fettanhang der Ratte mit Hilfe markierter Glukose. II. Experimentelle und klinische Erfahrungen (Determination of blood insulin in the epididymal fat appendage of the rat with the aid of labelled glucose. II. Experimental and clinical results). *Klin. Wochenschr.*, 37:1239–1244.
42. Pfeiffer, E. F., Ditschuneit, H., and Schöffling, K. (1959): Clinical and experimental studies of insulin secretion following tolbutamide and metahexamide administration. *Ann. N.Y. Acad. Sci.*, 82:479–486.
43. Pfeiffer, E. F., Ditschuneit, H., and Schöffling, K. (1961): Über die Bestimmung von Insulin im Blut am epididymalen Fettanhang der Ratte mit Hilfe markierter Glukose. IV. Die Dynamik der Insulin-sekretion des Stoffwechselgesunden und des Altersdiabetikers nach wiederholter Belastung mit Glukose, Sulfonylharnstoffen und menschlichem Wachstumshormon, ein Beitrag zur Pathogenese des menschlichen Altersdiabetes (Determination of blood insulin in the epididymal fat appendage of the rat with the aid of labelled glucose. IV. The dynamics of insulin secretion in healthy subjects and maturity-onset diabetics after repeated loading with glucose, sulphonylureas and human growth hormone. A contribution to our knowledge of the pathogenesis of human maturity-onset diabetes). *Klin. Wochenschr.*, 39:415–430.
44. Pfeiffer, E. F., and Raptis, S. (1972): Controlled extension of oral antidiabetic therapy on former insulin dependent diabetics by means of the combined i.v. glibenclamide-glucose-response test. *Diabetologia*, 8:41–47.
45. Pfeiffer, E. F., Raptis, S., and Schröder, K. E. (1974): Die Bedeutung der einmaligen kombinierten i.v. Glibenclamid-Glucose-Belastung für Auswahl, Indikationsstellung und Prognose der Glibenclamidehandlung des sogenannten "insulinbedürftigen" Tolbutamid-resistenten Erwachsenendiabetes (The value of the one dose-combined i.v. glibenclamide-glucose tolerance test in the selection, establishment of indications and prognosis for glibenclamide treatment among patients with so-called "insulin-dependent" tolbutamide-resistant maturity-onset diabetes). *Dtsch. Med. Wochenschr.*, 90:1281–1294.
46. Pfeiffer, E. F., Steigerwald, H., Sandritter, W., Bänder, A., Mager, A., Becker, U., and Retiene, K. (1957): Vergleichende Untersuchungen von Morphologie und Hormongehalt des Kälberpankreas nach Sulfonylharnstoffen (D 680) (Comparative investigations of the morphology and hormone content of calf pancreas after administration of sulphonylureas (D 680)). *Verh. Dtsch. Ges. Inn. Med.*, 63:604–617.
47. Ponari, O., Civardi, E., Megha, S., Pini, M., Portioli, D., and Dettori, A. G. (1979): Anti-platelet effects of long-term treatment with gliclazide in diabetic patients. *Throm. Res.*, 16:191–203.
48. Prince, M. J., and Olefsky, J. M. (1980): Direct in-vitro effect of a

sulfonylurea to increase human fibroblast insulin receptors. *J. Clin. Invest.*, 66:608–611.
49. Raptis, S. (1975): Pro und Kontra der oralen Diabetes Therapie (For and against oral diabetes therapy). 35:4537–4542.
50. Raptis, S. (1972): 15 Jahre Orale Diabetes-Therapie (Fifteen years of oral diabetes therapy). *Dtsch. Med. J.*, 23:617–624.
51. Raptis, S: Orale Antidiabetika der 1. und 2. Generation (Oral antidiabetics of the first and second generations). *Münch. Mediz. Wochenschr.*, 40:1836–1837.
52. Raptis, S.: Insulinsekretion unter normalen und pathologischen Bedingungen. Neue Möglichkeiten der oralen Diabetes-therapie mit Sulfonylharnstoffen der 2. Generation (Insulin secretion under normal and abnormal conditions. New potentialities of oral diabetes therapy with sulphonylureas of the second generation). In: *Moderne Diabetologie -Aktuelle Problematik und Trendanalyse.* V. Symposium in Sanderbusch, 5 May 1973, Tagungsband 25–47.
53. Raptis, S., Dimitriadis, G., Karaiskos, K., Rosenthal, J., Zoupas, C., and Moulopoulos, S. (1980): Long term effects of an α-glucosidase inhibitor on catecholamine levels and insulin requirements as assessed by the artificial beta-cell. 40th Annual Meeting American Diabetes Assoc. *Diabetes, (Suppl.* 2) 29:163.
54. Raptis, S., Laube, H., Katsilambros, N., Hinz, M., Rothmann, G., and Pfeiffer, E. F. (1974): Tierexperimentelle und klinische Untersuchungen mit dem neuen Sulfonylharnstoff Glisoxepid (BS 4231) (Animal experiments and clinical studies with the new sulphonylurea glisoxepide (BS 4231)). Prodiaban-Symposium, Berlin, December 1973, Schattauer-Verlag Stuttgart, 73–82.
55. Raptis, S., Loeprecht, H., Schlegel, W., Lehmann, E., Röventrunck, U., Rosenthal, J., Hrstka, V., and Schmidt, F. H. (1977): Modulation of insulin, C-peptide, gastrin, secretin, pancreozymin release and blood glucose concentration in portal and peripheral blood following glibenclamide in man. *Diabetologia*, 13:426–427.
56. Raptis, S., and Pfeiffer, E. F. (1971): Sulfonylharnstoffe als orale Antidiabetika der 1. und 2. Generation (Sulphonylureas as oral antidiabetics of the first and second generations). *Therapie-Woche*, 21:8 578–589.
57. Raptis, S., and Pfeiffer, E. F. (1971): Sulfonylharnstoffe als orale Antidiabetika der 1. und 2. Generation (Sulphonylureas as oral antidiabetics of the first and second generations). *Therapiewoche*, 21:578–590.
58. Raptis, S., Rau, R. M., Schröder, K. E., Faulhaber, J. D., and Pfeiffer, E. F. (1969): Comparative study of insulin secretion following repeated administration of glucose, tolbutamide and glibenclamide (HB 419) in diabetic and non-diabetic human subjects. *Horm. Metab. Res. (Suppl.)*, 1:65–72.
59. Raptis, S., Rothenbuchner, G., and Pfeiffer, E. F. (1971): Fortschritte in der Diabetes Therapie (Advances in diabetes therapy). *Wien. Med. Wochenschr.* 14:261–269.
60. Raptis, S., Rothenbuchner, G., Schröder, K. E., and Pfeiffer, E. F. (1973): Möglichkeiten und Grenzen der modernen Tablettentherapie (Potentialities and limitations of modern tablet therapy). *Therapie-Woche*, 23:936–944.

61. Raptis, S., Schröder, K. E., and Pfeiffer, E. F. (1973): Die kombinierte intravenöse Glukose-Glibenclamid-Belastung als Test zur Vorhersage der Erfolges der oralen Dauerbehandlung des Diabetes der Erwachensen mit Glibenclamid (The combined intravenous glucose-glibenclamide tolerance test for predicting the success of long-term oral treatment of maturity-onset diabetics with glibenclamide). 79. Tagung der Deutschen Ges, f. Inn. Med., Wiesbaden 29 April - 3 Mai 1973, Bergmann-Verlag, München 1210–1213.
62. Reddi, A. S., Oppermann, W., and Velasco, C., Camerini-Davalos, R. A. (1978): Diabetic microangiopathy in KK mice. V. effect of early glyburide treatment on kidney glucosyltransferase activity. *Exp. Mol. Pathol.* 29:442–447.
63. Retiene, K., Petzoldt, R., Althoff-Zucker, C., Beyer, J., and Schöffling, K. (1969): Clinical studies on glibenclamide (HB 419). *Horm. Metab. Res. (Suppl.)* 1:55–60.
64. Rothenbüchner, G., Raptis, S., and Pfeiffer, E. F. (1971): Insulin oder orale Antidiabetika aus der Sicht von Forschung und Klinik (Insulin or oral antidiabetic from the standpoint of research and clinical practice). *Heilkunst,* 84:215–220.
65. Sachse, G., and Willms, B. (1979): Effect of the α-glucosidase-inhibitor BAY-g-5421 on blood glucose control of sulphonylurea-treated diabetics and insulin-treated diabetics. *Diabetologia,* 17:287–290.
66. Schmidt, D. D., Frommer, W., Müller, L., and Truscheit, E. (1979): Glucosidase-Inhibitoren aus Bazillen (Glucosidase inhibitors from bacilli). *Naturwissenschaften,* 66:584–589.
67. Schröder, K. E., Raptis, S., and Pfeiffer, E. F. (1975): Zur Frage des Versagens der Sulfonylharnstoffbehandlung bei sogenannten Erwachsenendiabetes (Failure of sulphonylurea treatment in so-called maturity-onset diabetes). 10. KongressDeutsch. Diabetes. Gesellschaft Ulm 1975 *Nov. Inf. Vortrag,* Nr. 62.
68. Stötter, G. (1970): Hypoglykämien nach Behandlung mit Glibenclamid (Euglucon^R 5). [Hypoglycaemic attacks after treatment with glibenclamide (Euglucon ^{R} 5)]. *Münch. Med. Wochenschr.,* 112:2192–2194.
69. Tranquada, R. E., Bernstein, S., and Martin, H. E. (1963): Irreversible lactic acidosis associated with phenphormin therapy. *J. Am. Med. Assoc.,* 184:37–46.
70. University Group Diabetes Program (1970): A study of the effects of hypoglycemia agents on vascular complications in patients with adult-onset diabetes: II. Mortality results. *Diabetes,* 19:789–810.
71. University Group Diabetes Program (1971): Effects of hypoglycemic agents on vascular complications in patients with adult-onset diabetes: IV. A preliminary report on Phenformin results. *J.A.M.A.* 217:777–798.
72. University Group Diabetes Program (1976): A study of the effects of hypoglycemic agents on vascular complications in patients with adult-onset diabetes. VI. Supplementary report on nonfatal events in patients treated with tolbutamide. *Diabetes,* 25:1129–1152.

The Importance of Islets of Langerhans for Modern Endocrinology, edited by K. Federlin and J. Scholtholt, Raven Press, New York © 1984.

Treatment of Diabetes Mellitus: Insulin

Karl Schöffling, Christoph Rosak, and Peter-Henning Althoff

Department of Endocrinology and Metabolism, Center of Internal Medicine, Johann Wolfgang Goethe University, D-6000 Frankfurt am Main, Federal Republic of Germany

In presenting this article, we are celebrating the 60th birthday of Ernst Pfeiffer. Several months ago, we commemorated the 60th anniversary of the discovery of insulin.

During July and August 1921, Banting and Best (3) gave their best crude pancreas extract to pancreatectomized dogs and for the first time observed a fall in blood glucose. The first human to receive this insulin preparation was Leonard Thompson, who responded well to this treatment. He received his first injection on January 11, 1922.

After these initial successes, a frustrating period followed, since many difficulties arose in obtaining adequate quantities of stable material. Jackson (12) described this situation in the last issue of the IDF-Bulletin, and we would like to quote a few of his sentences: "The principal difficulty in relation to the large-scale production of insulin lay in the development of extraction methods which would both maintain potency and achieve stability. Because it was known that enzymes, especially trypsin, destroyed the activity of insulin content of the pancreas, a way had to be found to overcome this problem. Prof. C. B. Collip overcame the problem by fractional precipitation, but between March and May 1922, no useable insulin was manufactured."

Before the discovery of insulin, ketoacidosis was the main cause of death in diabetics. The decrease in overall mortality from diabetic coma among all Joslin Clinic (25) patients is eloquently illustrated in Fig. 1. However, even among patients

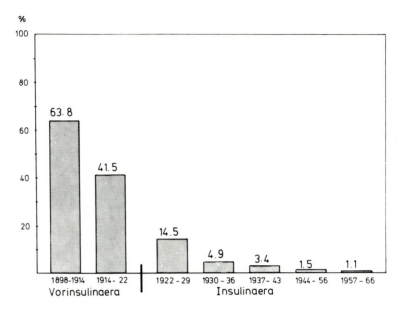

FIG. 1. Mortality of patients with Coma diabeticum in the Joslin Clinic between 1898 and 1961.

treated for ketoacidosis and coma in the insulin era, the mortality rate still varies roughly from 7.2% to 12.9% depending on which study is cited. The persistence of such a substantial mortality rate underscores the continuing clinical importance of diabetic coma and the vigilance required during therapy with respect to its precipitating causes such as infections, sepsis, myocardial infarction, thyroid storm, and immunological insulin resistance (4).

We last investigated these problems several years ago, and we observed between 20 and 40 comas per year in our hospital. Among these patients, 25% had coma as the first manifestation of diabetes, which demonstrates that current health education is still inadequate insofar as the recognition of type I diabetes is concerned.

After we learned from Turner in 1971 (27) how fast insulin disappears from the blood stream after i.v. infusion and after we saw the results of Alberti's group (1) in 1973, we stopped the 5-decade-old conventional way of treating diabetic ketoacidosis and switched to the so-called low-dose insulin regimen. The ideal approach appears to be, based on our own experience (2) and the results of others, the continuous intravenous infusion of a small dose of insulin via an infusion pump. Fig. 2 demonstrates that we need 4 to 8 units of regular insulin per hour in these eight patients to reduce blood glucose to an acceptable level. To avoid adhesion of insulin to glass and plastic tubing on the one hand, and to exclude on the other hand, the low risk of hepatitis associated with human serum albumin, we dissolved the insulin in Haemacel®.

Changes in blood glucose (Fig. 3), β-hydroxybutyric acid (Fig. 4), and osmolarity (Fig. 5) during such treatment in these patients demonstrate the effectiveness of this regimen. The advantage of this new method of treating diabetic ketoacidosis is that it significantly lowers the risk of hypoglycemia, hypokalemia and, possibly, cerebral edema.

The theoretical contribution of this new approach to treatment is that it refutes the 50-year-old concept of tremendous

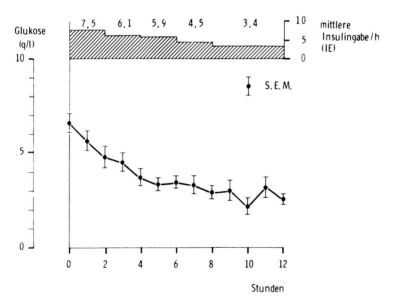

FIG. 2. Changes in blood glucose in patients with Coma diabeticum during low-dose insulin treatment.

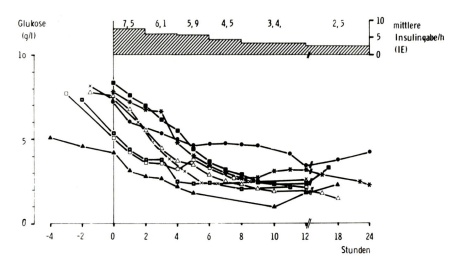

FIG. 3. Changes in blood glucose in eight patients with Coma diabeticum during low-dose insulin treatment.

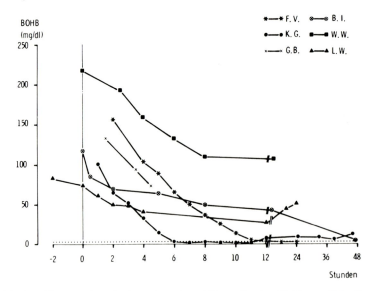

FIG. 4. Changes in β-hydroxybutyric acid in patients with Coma diabeticum during low-dose insulin treatment.

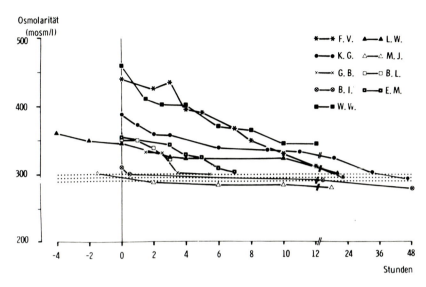

FIG. 5. Changes in osmolarity in patients with Coma diabeticum during low-dose insulin treatment.

insulin resistance in ketoacidosis. There is certainly insulin resistance in ketoacidosis, more so when diabetic ketoacidosis is associated with infection, but it is much less pronounced than has been assumed in the past (4).

Of the total population of diabetic patients, 20% require insulin treatment. This category includes type I diabetics regardless of age at onset, type II patients with hyperglycemia not responsive to dietary measures and/or sulfonylurea agents, and insulin-dependent diabetics during periods of intercurrent stress.

The most widely used insulin preparations, especially in the United States (5,8), are the intermediate-acting NPH and Lente insulins and the rapid-acting regular and semilente insulins. The situation in Germany and in other parts of Europe (19,20) is more complicated, as is evident in Fig. 6. Showing this graph brings to mind one famous sentence of Johann Wolfgang von Goethe from the ninth book of the *Xenien*: Amerika, du hast es besser, als unser Kontinent, der alte." But we have to live with this great variety, which also has some advantages. In Germany practically all insulins are purified; this means that they were subjected to gel chromatography. Many of them also are purified

170 INSULIN TREATMENT OF DIABETES

Präparat	Spezies	Wirkungsprofil	Spritz-Eß-Abst Min	Wirkg. max Std	Wirkg. dauer Std	Lsg./Susp	Bemerkung
Insulin Hoechst Insulin S Hoechst	R S		15-20	1-2	5-7	Lsg	
Novo-Actrapid	S		15-20	1-2	5-7	Lsg	
Insulin Leo	S		15-20	1-2	5-7	Lsg	
Komb-Insulin Komb-Insulin S Hoechst	R S		20-30	1½-4	9-14	Lsg	⅓ Normal-Insulin ⅔ Insulin-Surfen-Komplex
Insulin Novo Semilente	S		45-60	5-10	12-16	Susp	Zink-Insulin Komplex
Insulin Initard Leo	S		30	3-5	12-18	Susp	½ Normal-Insulin ½ NPH-Insulin
Depot-Insulin Hoechst Depot-Insulin S Hoechst	R S		30-45	3-6	10-16	Lsg	Insulin-Surfen-Komplex
Insulin Novo Rapitard	R+S		30	4-12	14-18	Susp	¼ Normal-Insulin ¾ Insulinkristalle
HG-Insulin HG-Insulin S Hoechst	R S		45	3-7	12-16	Lsg	Humanglobin-insulin
Insulin Mixtard Leo	S		30-45	3-7	14-20	Susp	30% Normal-Insulin 70% NPH-Insulin
Insulin Novo Monotard	S		45-60	6-14	18-22	Susp	30% amorph 70% Kristallinsulin
Insulin Retard NPH Leo	S		45-60	6-10	16-22	Susp	Protamin-Insulin-Kristalle
Long-Insulin Hoechst	S		60	3-8	18-26	Susp	Kristall + amorph Insuline + Insulin-Surfen-Komplex
Insulin Novo Lente	R+S		60	7-14	über 24	Susp	30% amorph 70% Kristallinsulin
Insulin Novo Ultralente	R		60	10-30	über 34	Susp	Zink-Insulin-Komplex

FIG. 6. Insulin preparations in Germany, 1982.

by ion exchange chromatography. Most of the insulins in Germany are monospecies insulins (the only exceptions today are Lente and Rapitard).

New German insulins, which were introduced in 1981 and 1982, are the so-called Des-Phe insulins (Fig. 7), with the trade name Optisulin®. These insulins, produced semisynthetically be cleaving phenylalanine in position 1 of the B chain, have the same biological activity as normal insulin, but the new physicochemical properties permit the production of stable monospecies

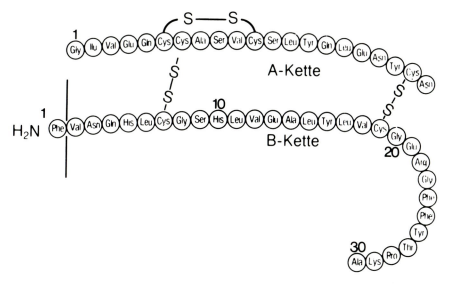

FIG. 7. Des-Phe-Insulin Optisulin R®.

combination insulins. Results of our first study in five clinics (24) demonstrate (Table 1) that these preparations are new intermediary insulins with a marked initial effect and a balanced relation between initial action and depot action and with some advantages in comparison with Surfen insulin, the preparation that up to now has been most widely used in Germany.

The preparation of human insulin by recombinant DNA technology became a reality in 1979, as first described by Goeddel and co-workers (10). The new technology has now made possible the production of biosynthetic human insulin by processes that are commercially feasible, thereby effectively precluding the worldwide insulin shortage forecast for the 1990s (23).

Today it is also possible to produce human insulin from pork insulin, which differs by only one amino acid in position B 30. Porcine insulin can be converted to human insulin by enzymatic synthesis, in which alanine is removed by carboxypeptidase A and threonine coupled by trypsin (15).

In our first study using human insulin, we investigated the influence of three human insulins (BHI Lilly, SSI Novo, Hoechst 11 H) on glucose and other metabolic substrates and compared

TABLE 1. Mittelwerte der Blutzuckerparameter

Blutzucker (mg/dl)	Depot-Insulin	Hoe 03 R$_{20}$	Hoe 03 R$_{25}$	Depot-Insulin	Behandlungs-unterschiede
NBZ	152	163	154	152	n.s.
MAX-NBZ	72.9	53.4	52.7	71.3	$p < 0.05$
NBZ-MIN	4.9	7.5	9.7	9.2	n.s.
NBZ-NACHM.BZ	−18.2	−39.4	−27.1	−5.2	n.s.
|NBZ-NACHM.BZ|	58.8	71.7	72.9	68.6	n.s.
MBG	172.5	193.9	178.7	167.2	$p < 0.05$
ABEND-BZ-NACHM.BZ	20.5	10.8	20.2	21.3	n.s.

these results with those of tests employing these manufacturers analogous purified pork insulins as well as with the Pork-Des-Phe-Insulin Hoechst (17). Eight healthy male volunteers took part in this study. The different insulins were administered intravenously at a dosage of 0.075 U/kg as bolus. The observation period lasted over 3 hr, during which eight samples were drawn. No significant difference between the three human insulins and the three pork insulins were found in this study. In addition, the rise of blood glucose after Des-Phe insulin did not differ from that seen with the other preparations (Fig. 8). On the other hand, we observed a slightly more pronounced antilipolytic activity with the biosynthetic human insulin that with the PPI, which we did not observe in testing the semisynthetic insulins (Fig. 9). Also, blood levels of β-hydroxybutyric acid after BHI were in a lower range than after PPI (Fig. 10).

Having found these discrete differences in the antilipolytic and antiketogenic activity of biosynthetic human insulin, we became interested in the hormonal counterregulatory response to hypoglycemia after the different insulin types. Therefore, in a second study, we investigated (26) the secretion pattern of different hormones after insulin-induced hypoglycemia. Again, eight healthy male volunteers received 0.075 U/kg of purified pork insulin (PPI) i.v. and biosynthetic human insulin (BHI), respectively, both produced by the Eli Lilly Company. Blood samples were drawn eight times during 3 hr. Following the application of PPI and BHI, the blood glucose concentration (Fig. 11) declines to a nadir of 25.1 ± 3.7 mg/dl for PPI and 26.3 ± 2.9 mg/dl for BHI after 25 min. Thereafter, a slow, steady rise in blood glucose occurs, reaching baseline levels at the end of the study after 180 min.

After BHI-induced hypoglycemia, glucagon (Fig. 12) as well as adrenalin (Fig. 13) and cortisol (Fig. 14) show the same secretion patterns as after PPI injection. The cortisol result is in contrast to the results of Raptis et al. (16). They found higher cortisol values after BHI, but they used another insulin dosage. The growth hormone secretion (Fig. 15) pattern is similar following both insulins. However, the peak level at 60 min. is higher for BHI with 37 ng/ml compared to 27 ng/ml with PPI. This difference is not significant.

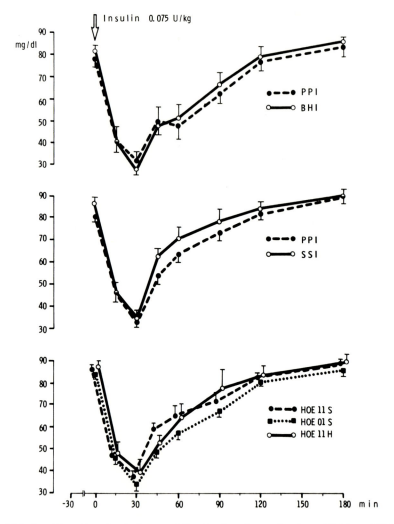

FIG. 8. Blood levels of glucose following insulin application of BHI and PPI (Lilly), SSI and PPI (Novo), Hoe 11 H, Hoe 11 S, and Hoe ol S (Hoechst) in eight volunteers. ($\bar{x} \pm$ S. E. M.)

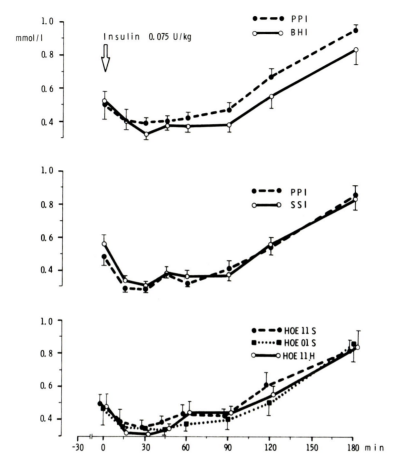

FIG. 9. Blood levels of free fatty acids following insulin application of BHI and PPI (Lilly), SSI and PPI (Novo), Hoe 11 H, Hoe 11 S, and Hoe ol S (Hoechst) in eight volunteers. ($\bar{x} \pm$ S. E. M.)

A completely different secretion pattern can be detected in prolactin secretion following PPI and BHI (Fig. 16). Following PPI, there is a gradual rise from the initial level 7.3 to 13.7 ng/ml at 45 min. and 13 ng/ml at 60 min. followed by a low decrease to values lower than starting point levels at 180 min. Following BHI, no rise in prolactin secretion could be detected.

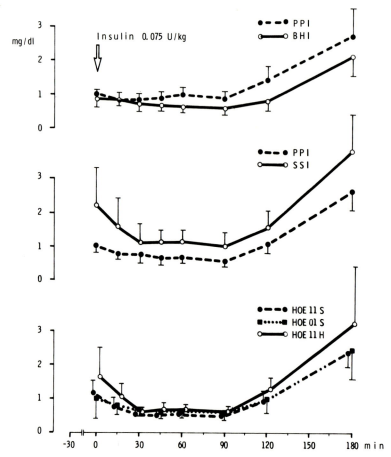

FIG. 10. Blood levels of β-hydroxybutyrate following insulin application of BHI and PPI (Lilly), SSI and PPI (Novo), Hoe 11 H, Hoe 11 S, and Hoe ol S (Hoechst) in eight volunteers. ($\bar{x} \pm$ S. E. M.)

The two insulins investigated in this study exhibit equal and comparable hypoglycemic effects; however, the secretion pattern of two of the counterregulatory hormones was different. Secretion of growth hormone after BHI was also studied by Raptis et al. (16) and by Federlin et al. (7). Their results are somewhat different from ours, but all these investigations, including our own, did not show significant differences in growth hormone secretion. So far as we know, no data on prolactin

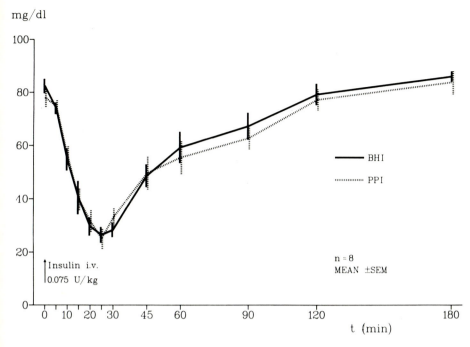

FIG. 11. Blood levels of glucose following insulin application of BHI and PPI (Lilly).

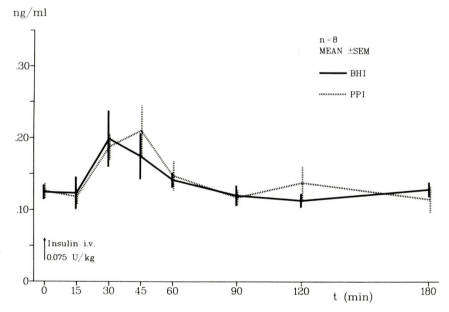

FIG. 12. Blood levels of glucagon following insulin application of BHI and PPI (Lilly).

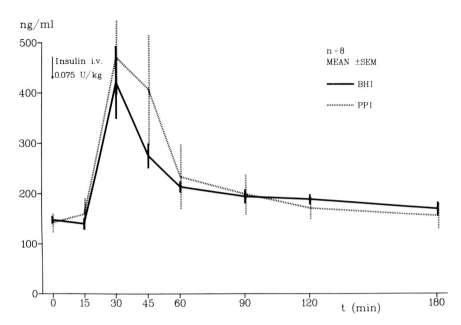

FIG. 13. Blood levels of adrenalin following insulin application of BHI and PPI (Lilly).

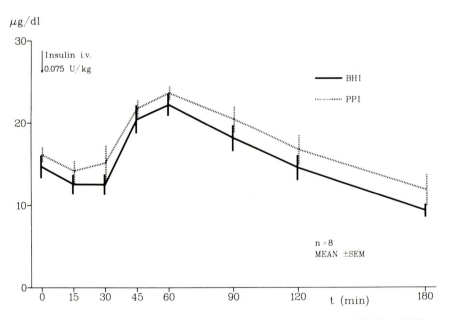

FIG. 14. Blood levels of cortisol following insulin application of BHI and PPI (Lilly).

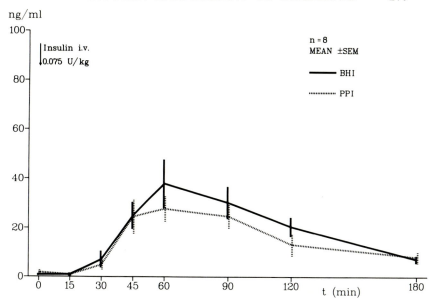

FIG. 15. Blood levels of growth hormone following insulin application of BHI and PPI (Lilly).

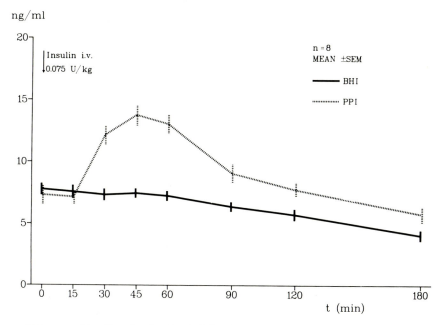

FIG. 16. Blood levels of prolactin following insulin application of BHI and PPI (Lilly).

secretion following BHI hypoglycemia are available today. In contrast to the hypoglycemia after PPI, no secretion of prolactin was detectable after BHI.

The basal hypothalamus also is involved in the regulation of prolactin secretion by producing prolactin inhibiting factor (PIF), which is thought to be dopamine. Dopamine stimulation reduces prolactin secretion and, conversely, enhances growth hormone secretion. The results presented can be explained by central dopamine stimulation by the homologous insulin BHI. Since prolactin is a potential diabetogenic stress hormone, the fact that BHI induces no prolactin secretion may be of clinical importance in the long-term treatment of diabetics.

The biosynthetic and semisynthetic human insulins are now available worldwide to many diabetologists (11,13,21). A great number of the early studies with BHI were published 1981 in *Diabetes Care*, edited by Skyler and Raptis (21). In Germany the registration of BHI-Regular was introduced very recently. The report contains 42 studies with 114 probands and 250 patients from seven different countries.

Certain observations suggest that BHI may be able to provide better glycemic control during treatment of insulin-dependent diabetes than can be achieved with the other insulin preparations (9). However, BHI appears to offer no general advantage in terms of preventing the immunological problems of this hormone treatment. In the report to the Bundesgesundheitsamt, antibody binding of BHI was found in 6% of the patients.

Insulin has now been available for 60 years in its regular form and for 40 years in the different intermediate and long-acting forms, and it is a truism that it does not "cure" diabetes in the sense that regular treatment with thyroxine cures hypothyroidism, leading to a normal life span and absence of complications (22). Insulin treatment, as generally implemented over the past 60 years, has merely postponed an early death from ketoacidosis without preventing the development of microvascular complications and premature atherosclerosis.

Many studies that were published during the last 8 years now give compelling evidence that good blood glucose control does prevent microvascular complications. We want to mention in this context only the study by Lauvaux and Pirart (14) and the long-term observations of Constam (6). If we accept these and many other epidemiological results, the aim of our treatment in the future must be a serious attempt to obtain blood glucose levels as close as possible to those in the nondiabetic. These epidemiological results and the experiences with closed- and open-loop insulin infusion systems have taught us that the most important consideration in insulin therapy is individualization of insulin doses and that, by providing the appropriate amount of insulin at the appropriate time, near normalization of glycemic control can be achieved in most patients (9).

Our present conception of a good control in a type I diabetic is summarized in Table 2. In most patients of this type, achieving this objective requires more than one insulin injection per day and more than a few blood tests during the day. Type I diabetes differs from many other chronic diseases in that the patient must be an active and knowledgeable partner in his own management. Doctors can suggest the best insulin and dietary regimens but, in the final analysis, it is the patient himself who must implement them (22). The patient's ability and willingness to comply depends on education, motivation, and training in self-control, psychological state, and patient-doctor relationship. Permanent and exact self-monitoring is an essential precondition for good control of a type I diabetic. Methods to establish such self-control have been improved in the past few years.

Diabur 5000, a new test strip for estimation of urinary glucose has some advantages over the older methods. In my opinion,

TABLE 2. *Good control in type I diabetes*

Blood glucose	
fasting	<130 mg/dl
1 hr p.p.	<180 mg/dl
2 hr p.p.	<160 mg/dl
3 hr p.c.	<130->90 mg/dl
HbA_1	<10%
Urine glucose	<5 g/24hr
Ketonuria	0
Cholesterol	<250 mg/dl
Triglycerides	<150 mg/dl
Body weight	<100% Broca

this technique should now replace the Clinitest method. The new strip was compared with the hexokinase method in our department in 379 tests (Fig. 17). The results of a multicenter study with 2540 tests (Fig. 18) were summarized at a meeting last year in Amsterdam. By combining test ranges, glucose concentrations of up to 5% can be detected by the strip test. False estimations of more than a one-color step do not occur. In our opinion, this method seems to be the best approach to urine testing in type I diabetics.

Blood glucose testing is equally necessary in the insulin-dependent diabetic. Reflectometers are the best devices, but they are quite expensive. We try to use them in pregnant diabetics, in patients with an open-loop insulin infusion system, and in

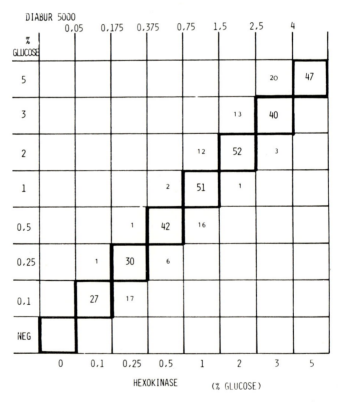

FIG. 17. Comparison of Diabur 5000 with the Hexokinase method (n = 379).

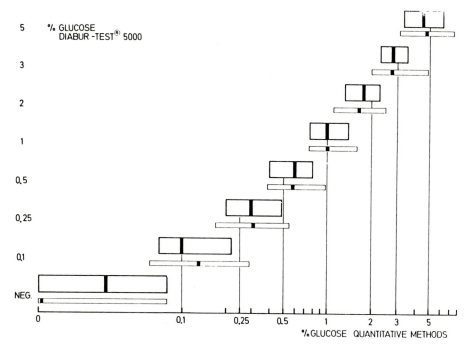

FIG. 18. Comparison of Diabur 5000 with methods for the quantitative determination of urinary glucose (laboratory tests). The 80% range (between 10th and 90th percentile) and the median are indicated. *Broad blocks*: Comparison with the HK-G6P-DH and Glud-DH® methods (n = 3,247). *Narrow blocks*: Comparison with the GOD methods (n = 858).

patients who can be termed brittle. During the last year, we have had good experiences with the glucometer manufactured by the Ames Company.

In a multicenter study involving nine clinics, blood glucose self-monitoring with the Haemoglukotest 20-800 was compared with the results of parallel samples taken by the patient with glucoquant and analyzed in the lab. 69% of the values read by the patients were correct. Below 200 mg/dl the mean deviation of the two corresponding values was ± 15 mg/dl (Fig. 19). In the same study, self-sampling of blood by the patients with glucoquant (Fig. 20)—another method of blood glucose control—was verified by parallel blood sampling by the technician and subse-

Haemo-Glukotest 20–800, Glucose [mg/dl] \ Profiliset für Gluco-quant, Glucose [mg/dl]	0–30	31–60	61–100	101–150	151–210	211–320	321–600	Σ
321–600						12	26	38
211–320					28	198	59	287
151–210		1	3	65	260	138	7	473
101–150		18	35	245	91	4		376
61–100	1		166	79	2	2		267
31–60	2	58	61	1				121
0–30	3	2	1					5
Σ	3	79	266	391	381	355	92	1567

FIG. 19. Comparison of Haemoglukotest 20–800 (patient) and Hexokinase (Laboratorium).

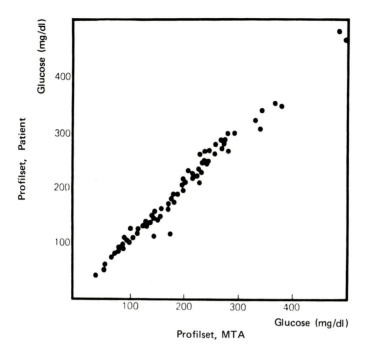

FIG. 20. Comparison of the glukoquant method between the patient and the technician.

quent glucose determination in the lab. A close correlation between the results was obtained. The mean deviation of the two corresponding values was ± 5.3% over the whole range of glucose concentrations.

We will conclude with a new closed loop-system, presented recently by Tattersall (22) (Fig. 21). Successful insulin treatment depends, like a watch, on a series of interconnected cogs; failure of any one of which will stop the watch. Blood glucose meters and infusion pumps do not liberate patients but bring them increased responsibilities. Conventional insulin treatment with subcutaneous injections, which will remain the primary mode of treatment in the majority of type I diabetics, has for the most part failed because it has never been tried enthusiastically enough.

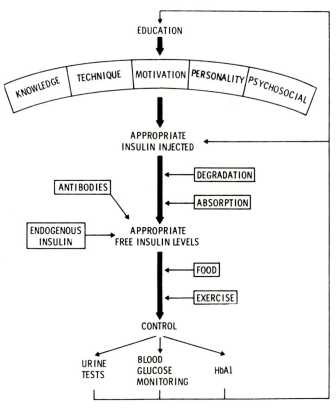

FIG. 21. The diabetic patient—a closed loop. (From Tattersall, ref. 22, with permission)

REFERENCES

1. Alberti, K. G. M. M., Hockaday, T. R. D., and Turner, R. C. (1973): Small doses of intramuscular insulin in the treatment of diabetic "coma." *Lancet*, 2:515.
2. Althoff, P. H., Neubauer, M., Petzoldt, R., and Schöffling, K. (1976): Behandlung des Coma diabeticum mit kleinen Insulin-mengen. *Verh. Dtsch. Ges. Inn. Med.*, 82:760.
3. Banting, F. G., and Best, C. H. (1922): The internal secretion of the pancreas. *J. Lab. Clin. Med.*, 7:251.
4. Baruh, S., Sherman, L., and Markowitz, S. (1981): Diabetic ketoacidosis and coma. *Med. Clin. North Am.*, 65:117.
5. Bressler, R., and Johnson, D. G. (1982): *Management of Diabetes mellitus*. John Wright, Boston.
6. Constam, C. R. (1977): Sind die diabetische Angio- und Neuropathie vermeidbar? *Med. Klin.*, 72:695

7. Federlin, K., Laube, H., and Velcovsky, H. G. (1981): Biologic and immunologic in vivo and in vitro studies with biosynthetic human insulin. *Diabetes Care*, 4:170.
8. Felig, P., Baxter, J. D., Broadus, A. E., and Frohman, L. A. (1981): *Endocrinology and Metabolism*. McGraw-Hill, New York.
9. Gerich, J. E. (1981): An appraisal of the role of biosynthetic human insulin in the future treatment of diabetes mellitus. *Diabetes Care*, 4:262.
10. Goeddel, D. V., Kleid, D. G., Bolivar, F., Heyncker, H. L., Yansura, D. G., Crea, R., Hirose, T., Kraszewski, A., Itakura, K., and Riggs, A. D. (1979): Expression in Escherichia coli of chemically synthesized genes for human insulin. *Proc. Natl. Acad. Sci. USA*, 76:106.
11. Hansen, B., Lernmark, A., Nielsen, J. H., Owerbach, D., and Welinger, B. (1982): New approaches to therapy and diagnosis of diabetes. *Diabetologia*, 22:61.
12. Jackson, J. G. L. (1982): Insulin: 1922–1982. *IDF-Bulletin*, 27:9.
13. Keen, H. (1982): Human insulin. 29. Postgraduate Course, ADA, January 25–27. Orlando, Florida.
14. Lauvaux, J. P., and Pirart, J. (1974): Diabetic retinopathy: a statistical study in 4400 diabetics. Relation to duration and control. *Diabetologia*, 10:383.
15. Morihara, K., Oka, T., and Tsuzuki, H. (1979): Semi-synthesis of human insulin by trypsin-catalysed replacement of Ala - B 30 by Thr in porcine insulin. *Nature*, 280:412.
16. Raptis, S., Karaiskas, C., Enzmann, F., Hatzidakis, D., Zoupas, C., Souvatzoglou, A., Diamantopoulos, E., and Mouloupoulos, S. (1981): Biologic activities of biosynthetic human insulin in healthy volunteers and insulin-dependent diabetic patients monitored by the artificial endocrine pancreas. *Diabetes Care*, 4:155.
17. Rosak, C., Althoff, P. H., and Schöffling, K. (1981): Synthese- und strukturmodifizierte Insuline. Untersuchungen zur biologischen Wirksamkeit. 1. Internat. Symposium: Neue Insuline, December 4–5, 1981. Freiburg, Germany.
18. Schöffling, K., Petzoldt, R., Walther, A., and Träbert, C. (1971): Epidemiologie, Ätiologie und Prognose des Coma diabeticum. In: *Biochemie und Klinik des Insulinmangels*. Thieme, Stuttgart.
19. Schöffling, K., and Müller, R. (1971): Die klinische Wirkung der Insulin-Zubereitungen. *Handbuch der experimentellen Pharmakologie*, Band 32/1 Insulin, Hrsg. E. Dörzbach, Springer-Verlag, Berlin.
20. Schöffling, K., and Schulz, F. (1974): Die Behandlung des Diabetes mellitus mit Insulin. In: *Diabetologie in Klinik und Praxis*, Hrsg. H. Mehnert and K. Schöffling. Thieme, Stuttgart.
21. Skyler, J. S., Pfeiffer, E. F., Raptis, S., and Viberti, G. C. (1981): Biosynthetic human insulin: progress and prospects. *Diabetes Care*, 4:140.
22. Tattersall, R. (1982): Intensive conventional therapy of IDDM. 29. Postgraduate Course, ADA, January 25–27. Orlando, Florida.
23. WHO Expert Committee on Diabetes mellitus: Second Report (1980): Technical Report Series No. 646. WHO, Geneva.
24. Zoltobrocki, M., Enzmann, F., Vanderbeke, O., Federlin, K., Laube, H., Klein, W., Valdenaire, K., Sauer, H., Riedesel, G., Schöffling, K.,

Neubauer, M., Willms, B., and Ahlhausen, S. (1980): Erste kontrollierte Multizenterstudie zur Erfassung des Wirkprofils einer neuartigen Insulinzubereitung mit Des-Phe-Insulin. *Akt. Endokrinol.*, 1:41.
25. Bradley, R. F. (1971): Diabetic ketoacidosis and coma. In: *Joslin's Diabetes mellitus*. Lea and Febiger, Philadelphia.
26. Rosak, C., Althoff, P. H., and Schöffling, K. (1982): Reduced prolactin response to human insulin-induced hypoglycemia—a possible unique advantage over pork insulin. 42nd annual meeting, ADA., June 13–15. San Francisco.
27. Turner, R. C., Grayburn, J. A., Newman, G. B., and Nabarro, J. D. N. (1971): Measurement of the insulin delivery rate in man. *J. Clin. Endocrinol.*, 33:279.

The Importance of Islets of Langerhans for Modern Endocrinology, edited by K. Federlin and J. Scholtholt, Raven Press, New York © 1984.

Artificial Endocrine Pancreas and Portable Insulin Pumps: Effect of Improved Glucose Control on Hormonal and Metabolic Abnormalities and the Development of Microvascular Complications in Type I Diabetes

Wolfgang Kerner

Department of Internal Medicine I, University of Ulm, D 7900 Ulm, Federal Republic of Germany

Despite considerable scientific effort, the pathogenesis of diabetic microvascular disease has not been elucidated up to now. There are mainly two controversial theories: (a) Inadequate control of blood glucose associated with metabolic and hormonal abnormalities by the currently employed "conventional" insulin therapy is the predominant pathogenetic factor; and (b) Development of diabetic complications is inherent to the disease and is unrelated to the quality of metabolic and hormonal control achieved by insulin administration. It is obvious that in proof of both theories "metabolic and hormonal abnormalities" must be eliminated. This is the point from which problems arise.

First, how can hormonal and metabolic parameters be normalized? From theoretical reasons, it seems obvious to aim at normal blood glucose concentrations as the guideline for insulin administration because glucose is the main regulator for insulin secretion under physiological conditions. But it has yet to be demonstrated that glucose-controlled insulin infusion restores metabolite and hormone concentrations to normal. These results might be obtained in short-term experiments. Second, if hormone and metabolite concentrations can be normalized in parallel to glucose, does this really prevent diabetic late complications? The answer to this question will only be possible in long-term experiments.

From these considerations, it becomes evident that blood glucose normalization has to be the starting point for all examinations. This has become possible during the last few years by the development of artificial insulin delivery devices. This chapter summarizes some of the results obtained with such systems regarding the effect of normalized or at least improved glucose control on hormone and metabolite concentrations as well as on the development of microvascular complications. Some results from our laboratory have been published previously (17,54,55).

ARTIFICIAL INSULIN DELIVERY SYSTEMS

Artificial Endocrine Pancreas (AEP)

In 1974 the independently working groups of Pfeiffer and Clemens in Ulm and Leibel and Albisser in Toronto published the first successful development of a glucose-controlled insulin infusion system (1,31,32), thus bringing the pioneering attempts of Kadish (13) to an impressive success. Both systems withdraw blood continuously for glucose determination and infuse insulin into a peripheral vein. Insulin infusion rates are calculated from glucose values by a microcomputer using an empirically derived algorithm. This algorithm considers not only actual glucose values (static control) but also their rates of change (differential control). The insulin infusion pump is automatically controlled by the microcomputer. The Ulm apparatus later became commercially available (Biostator®-GCIIS, Miles Lab., Elkhart, Indiana, USA).

Blood glucose normalization in diabetics with such an artificial endocrine pancreas is possible up to several days under various conditions (e.g., meal intake, oral glucose tolerance test, exercise). Besides application to diabetes therapy, artificial pancreas systems have proven to be extremely valuable in diabetes research (2,15–22,24,26,29,30,31–46).

Portable Insulin Infusion Pumps

Slama and co-workers in Paris reported in 1974 on the treatment of type I diabetes with a portable insulin pump (57). In their experiment, insulin was infused intravenously with a rather bulky pump. Meanwhile, not only pumps have been improved considerably with respect to size and handling, but also alternative routes of insulin administration (subcutaneous, intraperitoneal) have been examined (47,52). However, the mode of operation is still the same: insulin is infused at a constant basal rate while supplemental doses are supplied for meals. Despite the lack of feedback regulation by glucose determination, it is possible to regulate blood glucose in most of the diabetics treated with portable insulin pumps within "near normal" values resulting in HbA_1 concentrations in the upper normal range.

EFFECT OF IMPROVED GLUCOSE CONTROL ON COUNTERREGULATORY HORMONE CONCENTRATIONS

Growth Hormone

Most authors agree that mean diurnal growth hormone (GH) levels are higher in conventionally treated type I diabetics than in normal subjects (8,27). Furthermore, exaggerated GH responses to exercise and arginine infusion have been described (9,10,25).

We examined the effect of short-term glucose control for 86 hr with an artificial endocrine pancreas on GH levels in insulin-dependent diabetics. Under conventional therapy, mean daily GH levels amounted to 2,9 ± 0,2 ng/ml in these patients and did not change significantly during the third day of blood glucose normalization (2,8 ± 0,3 ng/ml) (Table 1). Similar observations were made by Hershcopf et al. (11) and Schiffrin et al. (53), who treated their patients with portable insulin pumps for 14 or 4 days and did not detect changes of GH concentrations. On the contrary, Tamborlane et al. (59) were able to reduce basal GH

TABLE 1. *Mean diurnal levels of blood glucose (BG), growth hormone (GH), glucagon (IRG) and cortisol in 8 normal subjects and 6 diabetics under conventional insulin therapy and during the third day of treatment with the AEP (Mean values ± SEM)*

	Normal subjects	Diabetics	
		Conventional treatment	AEP
BG (mg/dl)	79 ± 3	188 ± 25	97 ± 3
GH (ng/ml)	1.7 ± 0.3	2.9 ± 0.2	2.8 ± 0.5
IRG (pg/ml)	128 ± 19	260 ± 39	161 ± 22
Cortisol (μg/dl)	6.6 ± 0.6	6.3 ± 0.3	4.7 ± 0.5

levels after 2 weeks of pump treatment significantly to values similar to those of their controls.

Besides diurnal GH levels, we examined the response of this hormone to physical exercise and to arginine infusion. Patients undertook exercise tests (one in the morning, another in the afternoon) on a bicycle ergometer (75 watts for 45 min) while they were treated conventionally with insulin, and during the third day of blood glucose normalization. Arginine infusion tests (0.5 g/kg bodyweight within 30 min) were performed 12 and 86 hr after the start of treatment with the artificial pancreas.

Maximum increases in GH levels during the morning exercise test were of comparable size in diabetics on both forms of treatment and in normal subjects. Interestingly, during afternoon exercise, the increment of GH values was lower in conventionally treated diabetics than in the other groups (Table 2). There is no obvious explanation for this phenomenon. In contrast to these observations, Tamborlane et al. (59) reported on an exagerted increase of GH levels after exercise in conventionally treated diabetics that was normalized after 2 weeks of pump treatment. GH concentrations, in response to arginine, were elevated in our patients 12 hr after the start of blood glucose normalization, but returned to normal after 86 hr (Fig. 1).

Glucagon (IRG)

It is well known that IRG levels are abnormal in diabetics. Increased levels of this hormone have been described throughout the day (61) for the responses to arginine infusion (61) and

TABLE 2. *Responses of blood glucose (BG), growth hormone (GH) and free fatty acids (FFA) to exercise in 8 normal subjects and 6 diabetics under conventional therapy and during the third day of treatment with the AEP (Mean values ± SEM)*

	GH (ng/ml)		FFA (mmoles/liter)		BG (mg/dl)	
	Before exercise	Maximum increment	Before exercise	Maximum increment	Before exercise	Maximum change
Morning exercise (11.30–12.15)						
Normal subjects	1.3 ± 0.5	6.8 ± 1.4	0.40 ± 0.05	0.32 ± 0.08	76 ± 3	− 6 ± 1
Diabetics						
Conventional treatment	2.2 ± 1.3	8.6 ± 2.7	0.42 ± 0.05	0.18 ± 0.07	147 ± 21	−50 ± 11
AEP	3.1 ± 1.1	7.3 ± 3.3	0.40 ± 0.06	0.29 ± 0.06	93 ± 5	−23 ± 5
Afternoon exercise (17.30–18.15)						
Normal subjects	0.5 ± 0.1	5.1 ± 1.3	0.48 ± 0.08	0.36 ± 0.09	82 ± 4	−12 ± 3
Diabetics						
Conventional treatment	2.8 ± 1.7	2.3 ± 1.2	0.73 ± 0.11	0.40 ± 0.13	221 ± 43	−10 ± 9
AEP	2.7 ± 1.1	8.3 ± 3.8	0.35 ± 0.07	0.31 ± 0.06	96 ± 5	−14 ± 6

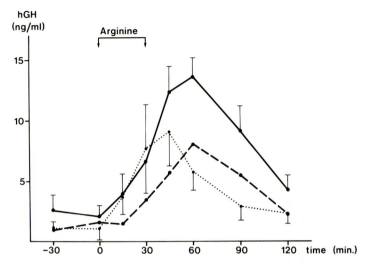

FIG. 1. Growth hormone (hGH) responses to intravenous arginine infusion in normal subjects (n = 8, - - -) and diabetics (n = 6) under control of the AEP for 12 (———) and 86 (. . . .) hr. (From Schock, ref. 55, with permission)

to glucose intake (28). On the contrary, IRG secretion during hypoglycemia seems to be diminished (6).

In our experiments, we were able to demonstrate a normalization of diurnal IRG concentrations at the third day of blood glucose normalization (see Table 1). Similarly, IRG responses to arginine infusion, which were still increased after 12 hr of treatment with the artificial pancreas, were normalized after 86 hr (Fig. 2). Similar results have been reported by others (12, 14,51). Regarding IRG responses to oral glucose, we were not able to restore a normal pattern despite perfect glucose control before (12 hr) and after (3 hr) glucose intake (17). In contrast to these results, Shichiri et al. (56) reported normalization of IRG levels in a comparable experiment. Finally, Ensinck et al. (5) and Bolli et al. (4) were not able to normalize glucagon secretion during hypoglycemia after 24 or 14 hr of treatment with an AEP.

Cortisol

In contrast to earlier reports (3,23), we did not detect any abnormalities of diurnal cortisol levels in conventionally treated

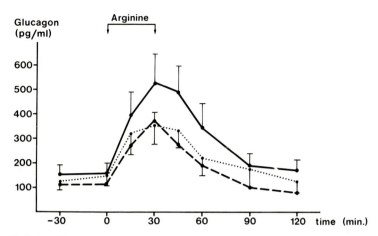

FIG. 2. Glucagon responses to intravenous arginine infusion in normal subjects (n = 8, ----) and diabetics (n = 6) under control of the AEP for 12 (———) and 86 hr (. . . .). (From Schock et al., ref. 55, with permission)

diabetics. This is in accordance with the findings of Schiffrin et al. (53) and Hershcopf et al. (11).

Catecholamines

Studies on catecholamines in type I diabetics were meager up to now. Tamborlane et al. (59) reported basal catecholamines concentrations to be normal in diabetics under conventional treatment. In these patients, exercised-induced increments of catecholamine levels were increased; they were normalized after 2 weeks of pump treatment. Zadik et al. (65) found that integrated catecholamine concentrations in diabetics were higher than in normal subjects, whereas Hershcopf et al. (11) from the same group could not detect this difference.

EFFECT OF IMPROVED GLUCOSE CONTROL ON METABOLITE, AMINO ACID, AND LIPID CONCENTRATIONS

Metabolites and Amino Acids

This subject has been extensively investigated by Zinman et al. (66) and Hanna et al. (7) under short-term glucose normalization with an AEP. These authors reported on a restoration of postmeal peaks of lactate and pyruvate under AEP control; however, postabsorptive concentrations of lactate and pyruvate were still increased. The elevated concentrations of free fatty acids under conventional insulin therapy were entirely normalized during AEP control, whereas beta-hydroxybutyrate concentrations were incompletely corrected. Responses of amino acids to blood glucose normalization were different. The concentrations of many amino acids were improved, but the concentrations of some were suppressed below normal, which might be due to the hyperinsulinemia inherent to AEP treatment.

In our group of patients, mean diurnal FFA concentrations in conventionally treated diabetics were slightly elevated above normal, and were lowered by AEP treatment, but differences were statistically not significant (Table 3). With respect to ergometer tests, elevated preexercise FFA levels in the afternoon and decreased FFA increments upon exercise in the morning, observed under subcutaneous insulin therapy, were normalized by AEP treatment (see Table 2).

Using portable insulin pumps, Tamborlane et al. (60) and Pickup et al. (48) examined the effect of improved glucose control on metabolite and amino-acid concentrations. They demonstrated a normalization of the levels of lactate, pyruvate, alanine, FFA, and branched-chain amino acids after a few days of pump treatment.

Lipids

Tamborlane et al. (60) reported on a reduction to normal of elevated triglyceride and cholesterol concentrations in conventionally treated diabetics after 14 days of pump treatment. Similar observations were made by Pietri et al. (50), who, additionally, observed a reduction of LDL-cholesterol levels in diabetics treated with pumps for 2 to 3 weeks. In the study of Hershcopf et al. (11), improvement of glucose control for 2 weeks with portable pumps resulted in a decrease of triglyceride, but not cholesterol levels.

In our patients, 3 days of AEP treatment reduced lipid concentrations only slightly (see Table 3), which might be due to the

TABLE 3. *Mean diurnal levels of blood glucose (BG), total cholesterol, triglycerides and free fatty acids (FFA) in 8 normal subjects and 6 diabetics under conventional insulin therapy and during the third day of treatment with the AEP (Mean values ± SEM)*

	Normal subjects	Diabetics	
		Conventional treatment	AEP
Cholesterol (mmoles/liter)	4.6 ± 0.2	4.0 ± 0.3	3.6 ± 0.3
Triglycerides (mmoles/liter)	1.2 ± 0.1	1.4 ± 0.2	1.1 ± 0.1
FFA (mmoles/liter)	0.56 ± 0.05	0.61 ± 0.09	0.47 ± 0.04
BG (mg/dl)	79 ± 3	175 ± 15	96 ± 3

fact that they were not elevated above normal under conventional insulin therapy.

EFFECT OF IMPROVED GLUCOSE CONTROL ON DIABETIC MICROVASCULAR COMPLICATIONS

At the present time, there are only a few reports on regression of microvascular disease in pump-treated type I diabetic patients. White et al. (63) described the case of a 20 year-old girl in whom early diabetic retinopathy reversed after 36 days of "constant normoglycemia." In a series of nine patients without proliferative retinopathy improvement of glucose control for 5 to 9 months resulted in eight patients in a decreased vitreous fluorescein accumulation (64). Comparable results were reported by the Steno Study Group (58).

Regression of diabetic nephropathy was studied by measurement of exercise-induced microalbuminuria and glomerular filtration rate (GFR) in pump-treated patients. It was shown that microalbuminuria is reduced after 2 to 3 weeks of improved glucose control (62). A reduction of GFR was observed after 4 months (58). Finally, nerve conduction velocity was used as a parameter for quantitative evaluation of diabetic neuropathy. Pietri et al. (49) were able to demonstrate an increase in motor nerve conduction velocity in median and peroneal nerves after 6 weeks with preprogrammed continuous subcutaneous insulin infusion.

CONCLUSIONS

There were two questions we put forth initially: (a) Are abnormalities of hormones and metabolites reversed by physiologic glucose control in type I diabetics? and (b) Can microvascular complications in these patients be prevented by improved glucose control? With respect to the first question, results are encouraging but not equivocal. Some hormones and metabolites are totally normalized, whereas others show at best a tendency toward normal. In the future, a definite answer to this question will be possible after several months of normoglycemia have elapsed. At present, complete normalization was not observed yet. Research on the influence of normoglycemia on diabetic complications is just in the beginning. Currently, we are looking with some success at the development of earliest lesions, but we are not sure if manifestation of clinical detectable complications is really preceeded by the lesions we examine. Years will elapse until the second question can be answered definitely.

ACKNOWLEDGMENTS

This work was supported by LVA Württemberg and Dotation Herbert Weishaupt e.V. The authors wishes to thank Mrs. Ilse Wollmann for her excellent technical and secretarial assistance.

REFERENCES

1. Albisser, A. M., Leibel, B. S., Ewart, T. G., Davidovac, Z., and Zingg, W. (1974): An artificial endocrine pancreas., *Diabetes*, 23:389–396.
2. Beischer, W., Schmid, M., Kerner, W., Keller, L., and Pfeiffer, E. F. (1978): Feedback inhibition of insulin in healthy and overweight subjects studied by use of an artificial endocrine pancreas. *Horm. Metab. Res. (Suppl.)*, 8:97–106.
3. Bolinger, R. E., Lukert, B. P., and Freeman, J. C. (1965): Adrenal function and plasma insulin activity in poorly regulated diabetics. *Am. J. Med. Sci.*, 250:629.
4. Bolli, G., Calabrese, G., DeFeo, P., Compagnucci, P., Zega, G., Angletti, G., Cartechini, M. G., Santeusanio, F., and Brunetti, P. (1982): Lack of glucagon response in glucose counter-regulation in type-I- (insulin-dependent) diabetics: absence of recovery after prolonged optimal insulin therapy. *Diabetologia*, 22:100–105.
5. Ensinck, J. W., and Kanter, R. A. (1980): Glucagon responses to hypoglycemia in type I diabetic men after 24-hour glucoregulation by glucose-controlled insulin infusion. *Diabetes Care*, 3:285–289.
6. Gerich, J. E., Langlois, M., Noacco, C., Karam, J. H., and Forsham, P. H. (1973): Lack of glucagon response to hypoglycemia in diabetes: evidence for an intrinsic pancreatic alpha-cell defect. *Science*, 182:171–173.
7. Hanna, A. K., Zinman, B., Nakhooda, A. F., Minuk, H. L., Stokes, E. F., Albisser, A. M., Leibel, B. S., and Marliss, E. F. (1980): Insulin, glucagon, and amino acids during glycemic control by the artificial pancreas in diabetic man. *Metabolism*, 29:321–332.
8. Hansen, A. P., and Johansen, K. (1970): Diurnal patterns of blood glucose, serum free fatty acids insulin, glucagon and growth hormone in normals and juvenile diabetics. *Diabetologia*, 6:27–33.
9. Hansen, A. P., (1970): Abnormal serum growth hormone response to exercise in juvenile diabetics. *J. Clin. Invest.*, 49:1467–1478.
10. Hansen, A. P. (1971): Normalization of growth hormone hyper-response to exercise in juvenile diabetes after "normalization" of blood sugar. *J. Clin. Invest.*, 50:1806–1811.

11. Hershcopf, R., Plotnick, L. P., Kaya, K., Benedict, G. W., Hadji-Georgopoulos, A., Margolis, S., and Kowarski, A. A. (1982): Short term improvement in glycemic control utilizing continuous subcutaneous insulin infusion: the effect on 24-Hour integrated concentrations of counterregulatory hormones and plasma lipids in insulin-dependent diabetes mellitus. *J. Clin. Endocrinol. Metab.*, 54:504–509.
12. Horwitz, D. L., Gonen, B., Jaspan, J. B., Langer, B. G., Rodman, D., and Zeidler, A. (1979): An "artificial beta cell" for control of diabetes mellitus: effect on plasma glucagon levels. *Clin. Endocrinol.*, 11:639–644.
13. Kadish, A. H. (1963): Automation control of blood sugar. A servomechanism for glucose monitoring and control. *Trans. Am. Soc. Artif. Organs*, 9:363–367.
14. Kawamori, R., Shichiri, M., Kikuchi, M., Yamasaki, Y., and Abe, H. (1980): Perfect normalization of excessive glucagon responses of intravenous arginine in human diabetes mellitus with the artificial beta-cell. *Diabetes*, 29:762–765.
15. Kerner, W., Thum, Ch., Tamás, Gy., Beischer, W., Clemens, A. H., and Pfeiffer, E. F. (1976): Attempts at perfect normalization of glucose tolerance test of severe diabetics by artificial beta cell. *Horm. Metab. Res.*, 8:256–261.
16. Kerner, W., Beischer, W., Tamás, Gy., Raptis, S., and Pfeiffer, E. F. (1977): Die Insulinbehandlung des entgleisten Diabetes mellitus mit einem Künstlichen endokrinen Pankreas. *Dtsch. Med. Wochenschr.* 102:1500–1505.
17. Kerner, W., and Pfeiffer, E. F. (1977): Glucagon secretion in diabetics during glucose-controlled insulin infusion. *Diabetologia*, 13:408.
18. Kerner, W., Beischer, W., Herfarth, W., and Pfeiffer, E. F. (1978): Application of an artificial endocrine pancreas in the management of the diabetic surgical patient. *Horm. Metab. Res. (Suppl.)*, 8:159–161.
19. Kerner, W., Beischer, W., Maier, V., and Pfeiffer, E. F. (1978): Influence of insulin infusion kinetics of an artificial beta cell on blood glucose control in insulin-dependent diabetics. *Horm. Metab. Res. (Suppl.)*, 8:71–80.
20. Kerner, W., Beischer, W., Heinze, E., Herfarth, Ch., and Pfeiffer, E. F. (1980): Continuous blood glucose monitoring and feedback controlled dextrose infusion with an artificial beta cell in the diagnosis and treatment of organic hyperinsulinism. In: *Current Views on Hypoglycemia and Glucagon*, edited by D. Andreani, P. J. Lefebvre, and V. Marks, pp. 241–257. Academic Press, London, New York, Toronto, Sydney, San Francisco.
21. Kerner, W., Moll, H., Beischer, W., and Pfeiffer, E. F. (1982): Importance of early postprandial increases of insulin infusion rates in diabetics treated intravenously with insulin. *Horm. Metab. Res. (Suppl.)*, 12:210–212.
22. Kerner, W., Schultz, M., Schock, D., and Pfeiffer, E. F. (1982): Variations of insulin requirements in insulin dependent diabetics for meals taken at different times of the day. *Horm. Metab. Res. (Suppl.)*, 12:228–230.

23. Klein, R., Weigand, F. A., Iunes, M., and Greenman, L. (1956): Corticoids in serum of children with treated diabetes mellitus. *Pediatrics*, 17:274–279.
24. Klier, M., Kerner, W., Torres, A. A., and Pfeiffer, E. F. (1981): Comparison of the biologic activity of biosynthetic human insulin and natural pork insulin in juvenile-onset diabetic subjects assessed by the glucose controlled insulin infusion system. *Diabetes Care*, 4:193–195.
25. Koncz, L., Soeldner, J. S., Balodimos, M. C., Boden, G., Gleason, R. E., and Younger, B. (1973): Human growth hormone secretion after double stimulation with arginine in normal and insulin-dependent diabetic women. *Diabetes*, 22:694–705.
26. Meissner, C., Thum, Ch., Beischer, W., Winkler, G., Schröder, K. E., and Pfeiffer, E. F. (1975): Antidiabetic action of somatostatin-assessed by the artificial pancreas. *Diabetes*, 24:988–996.
27. Molnar, G. D., Taylor, M. F., Langworthy, A., Fatourechi, V. (1972): Diurnal growth hormone and glucose abnormalities in unstable diabetics: studies of ambulatory fed subjects during continuous blood glucose analysis. *J. Clin. Endocrinol. Metab.*, 34:837–846.
28. Müller, W. A., Faloona, G. R., and Unger, R. H. (1971): The effect of experimental insulin deficiency in glucagon secretion. *J. Clin. Invest.*, 50:1992–1999.
29. Navascues, I., Kerner, W., Meissl, M., and Pfeiffer, E. F. (1981): Effect of acarbose on blood glucose control and insulin requirements in insulin dependent diabetics assessed by the artificial pancreas. In: *Proceedings of the First International Symposium on Acarbose*, Montreux, 1981, edited by W. Creutzfeldt, pp. 455–460. Excerpta Medica, Amsterdam, Oxford, Princeton.
30. Neuhaus, Ch., Kerner, W., Maier, V., and Pfeiffer, E. F. (1978): D-Trp^8-D-Cys^{14}-somatostatin-demonstration of its differential suppressive activity in juvenile diabetics. *Horm. Metab. Res. (Suppl.)*, 8:115–118.
31. Pfeiffer, E. F., Thum, Ch., and Clemens, A. H. (1974): The artificial beta cell: a continuous control of blood sugar by external regulation of insulin infusion (glucose controlled insulin infusion system). *Horm. Metab. Res.*, 6:339–342.
32. Pfeiffer, E. F., Thum, Ch., and Clemens, A. H. (1974): Die Künstliche Beta-Zelle. *Naturwissenschaften*, 61:455.
33. Pfeiffer, E. F., Thum, Ch., Beischer, W., and Clemens, A. H. (1975): Die Künstliche Beta-Zelle in Experiment und Klinik. *Verh. Dtsch. Ges. Inn. Med.*, 81:602–615.
34. Pfeiffer, E. F., Beischer, W., Kerner, W., Yoshioka, M., and Clemens, A. H. (1976): The artificial endocrine pancreas in clinical research. In: *Endocrinology*, Proceedings of the International Congress of Endocrinology, Hamburg, 1976, edited by V. H. T. James, pp. 579–587. Excerpta Medica, Amsterdam.
35. Pfeiffer, E. F., Beischer, W., Thum, Ch., and Clemens, A. H. (1976): Le Pancreas endocrine artificiel en clinique et en recherche. In: *Journées Annuelles de Diabétologie de l'Hôtel Dieu*, pp. 278–296. Flammarion., Paris.

36. Pfeiffer, E. F., Beischer, W., and Kerner, W. (1977): The artificial endocrine pancreas in clinical research. *Horm. Metab. Res. (Suppl.)*, 7:95–112.
37. Pfeiffer, E. F., Kerner, W., and Beischer, W. (1977): The artificial endocrine pancreas in clinical research and practice. In: *Diabetes*, Proceedings of the IX Congress of the International Diabetes Federation, New Delhi, 1976, edited by J. S. Bajaj, pp. 465–480. Excerpta Medica, Amsterdam, Oxford.
38. Pfeiffer, E. F., Kerner, W., and Beischer, W. (1977): The artificial endocrine pancreas: experimental research and clinical application. In: *XIVth International Congress of Therapeutics*, Montpellier (1977), pp. 59–78. L'Expansion Scientifique Francaise, Paris.
39. Pfeiffer, E. F., Kerner, W., Beischer, W., and Klier, M. (1978): Insulin treatment during diabetic coma with an artificial endocrine pancreas. *Horm. Metab. Res. (Suppl.)*, 8:150–155.
40. Pfeiffer, E. F., Kerner, W., Herfarth, Ch., and Clemens, A. H. (1978): Das Künstliche endokrine Pankreas in Experiment und Klinik. *Dt. Ärztebl.*, 75:547–554.
41. Pfeiffer, E. F., Meissner, C., Beischer, W., Kerner, W., Léfèbvre, P. J., Raptis, S., and Tamas, Gy. (1978): Antidiabetic action of somatostatin assessed by artificial beta-cell. *Metabolism (Suppl.)*, 1:1415–1426.
42. Pfeiffer, E. F. (1978): Significance of renormalization of blood glucose concentration in diabetes mellitus. *Horm. Metab. Res. (Suppl.)*, 7:2–8.
43. Pfeiffer, E. F. (1979): Feedback controlled and pre-programmed insulin infusions in research and treatment of diabetes mellitus. In: *Artificial Pancreas. Clinical Applications*, edited by P. Drouin, L. Mejean, and G. Debry, pp. 13–59. Doin Editeurs, Paris.
44. Pfeiffer, E. F., and Kerner, W. (1979): The impact of insulin infusion systems upon the theory and practice of diagnosis and treatment of diabetes mellitus. In: *Diabetes 1979*. Proceedings of the 10th Congress of the International Diabetes Federation, Vienna, 1979. edited by W. K. Waldhäusl, pp. 637–643. Excerpta Medica, Amsterdam, Oxford, Princeton.
45. Pfeiffer, E. F., and Kerner, W. (1981): The artificial endocrine pancreas: its impact on the pathophysiology and treatment of diabetes mellitus. *Diabetes Care*, 4:11–26.
46. Pfeiffer, E. F., and Kerner, W. (1981): Das Künstliche Pankreas: Entwicklung und Bedeutung für die Erforschung und Behandlung der Zuckerkrankheit. *Verh. Dtsch. Ges. Inn. Med.*, 87:1408–1428.
47. Pickup, J. C., Keen, H., Parsons, J. A., and Alberti, K. G. M. M. (1978): Continuous subcutaneous insulin infusion: an approach to achieving normoglycemia. *Brit. Med. J.*, 1:204–207.
48. Pickup, J. C., Keen, H., Parsons, J. A., Alberti, K. G. M. M., and Rowe, A. S. (1979): Continuous subcutaneous insulin infusion: improved blood-glucose and intermediary-metabolite control in diabetics. *Lancet*, 1255–1258.
49. Pietri, A., Ehle, A. L., and Raskin, P. (1980): Changes in nerve conduction velocity after six weeks of gluco-regulation with portable insulin infusion pumps. *Diabetes*, 29:668–671.

50. Pietri, A., Dunn, F. L., and Raskin, P. (1980): The effect of improved diabetic control on plasma lipid and lipoprotein levels. A comparison of conventional therapy and continuous subcutaneous insulin infusion. *Diabetes*, 29:1001–1005.
51. Raskin, P., Pietri, A., and Unger, R. (1979): Changes in glucagon levels after four to five weeks of glucoregulation by portable insulin infusion pumps. *Diabetes*, 28:1033–1035.
52. Schade, D. S., Eaton, R. P., Friedman, N. M., and Spencer, W. (1980): Intraperitoneal delivery of insulin by a portable microinfusion pump. *Metabolism*, 29:699–702.
53. Schiffrin, A., Colle, E., and Belmonte, M. (1980): Improved control in diabetes with continuous subcutaneous insulin infusion. *Diabetes Care*, 3:643–647.
54. Schock, D., Schultz, M., Kerner, W., Maier, V., and Pfeiffer, E. F. (1978): The effect of three days of blood glucose normalization by means of an artificial endocrine pancreas on the concentrations of growth hormone, glucagon and cortisol in juvenile diabetics. *Horm. Metab. Res. (Suppl.)*, 8:93–96.
55. Schock, D., Schultz, M., Kerner, W., Maier, V., and Pfeiffer, E. F. (1981): The influence of normoglycemia on serum concentrations of growth hormone, glucagon and free fatty acids in juvenile diabetics. In: *New Approaches to Insulin Therapy*, edited by K. Irsigler, K. N. Kunz, D. R. Owens, and H. Regal, pp. 211–218. MTP Press Ltd., Falcon House, Lancaster, England.
56. Shichiri, M., Kawamori, R., and Abe, H. (1979): Normalization of the paradoxic secretion of glucagon in diabetics who were controlled by the artificial beta cell. *Diabetes*, 28:272–275.
57. Slama, G., Hauteconverture, M., Assan, R., and Tchobroutsky, G. (1974): One to five days of continuous intravenous insulin infusion on severe diabetic patients. *Diabetes*, 23:732–738.
58. Steno Study Group (1982): Effect of 6 months of strict metabolic control on eye and kidney function in insulin-dependent diabetics with background retinopathy. *Lancet*, 1:121–123.
59. Tamborlane, W. V., Sherwin, R. S., Koivisto, V., Hendler, R., Genel, M., and Felig, P. (1979): Normalization of the growth hormone and catecholamine response to exercise in juvenile-onset diabetic subjects treated with a portable insulin infusion pump. *Diabetes*, 28:785–788.
60. Tamborlane, W. V., Sherwin, R. S., Genel, M., and Felig, P. (1979): Restoration of normal lipid and aminoacid metabolism in diabetic patients treated with a portable insulin-infusion pump. *Lancet*, 1:1258–1261.
61. Unger, R. H., Aguilar-Parada, E., Müller, W. A., and Eisentraut, A. M. (1970): Studies of pancreatic alpha-cell function in normal and diabetic subjects. *J. Clin. Invest.*, 49:837–848.
62. Viberti, G., Pickup, J. C., Bilous, R. W., Keen, H., Mackintosh, D. (1981): Correction of exercise-induced microalbuminuria in insulin-dependent diabetics after 3 weeks of subcutaneous insulin infusion. *Diabetes*, 30:818–823.

63. White, M. C., Kohner, E. M., Pickup, J. C., and Keen, H. (1981): Reversal of diabetic retinopathy by continuous subcutaneous insulin infusion: a case report. *Br. J. Ophtalmol.*, 65:307–311.
64. White, N. H., Waltman, S. R., Krupin, T., and Santiago, J. V. (1982): Reversal of abnormalities in ocular fluorophotometry in insulin-dependent diabetes after five to nine months of improved metabolic control. *Diabetes*, 31:80–85.
65. Zadik, Z., Kayne, R., Kappy, M., Plotnick, L. P., and Kowarski, A. A. (1980): Increased integrated concentration of norepinephrine, epinephrine, aldosterone and growth hormone in patients with uncontrolled juvenile diabetes mellitus. *Diabetes*, 29:655–658.
66. Zinman, B., Stokes, E. F., Albisser, A. M., Hanna, A. K., Minuk, H. L., Stein, A. N., Leibel, B. S., and Marliss, E. B. (1979): The metabolic response to glycemic control by the artificial pancreas in diabetic man. *Metabolism*, 28:511–518.

The Importance of Islets of Langerhans for Modern Endocrinology, edited by K. Federlin and J. Scholtholt, Raven Press, New York © 1984.

Pancreas-Islet Transplantation

K. F. Federlin and R. G. Bretzel

Medical Clinic and Policlinic III, Universität Giessen Federal Republic of Germany

As shown by several experimental and clinical studies in the past, total endocrine replacement therapy for insulin-dependent diabetes mellitus in experimental animals is possible by transplantation of pancreatic allografts or by transplantation of the islets of Langerhans as free grafts. The reason for these attempts rests on the hypothesis that perfect metabolic control may inhibit or stop the development of diabetic late complications as retinopathy, nephropathy, neuropathy, or other lesions of various organs. Transplantation of endocrine pancreatic tissue, therefore, has to answer two main questions: (a) Does it guarantee perfect metabolic control? and (b) Are late complications inhibited when perfect control can be achieved? During the last 10 years, many aspects of whole pancreas as well as of isolated islet transplantation have been investigated, and both techniques have been used in experimental animals and in humans. From these in our brief summary, only a few can be mentioned. We shall try to select those that perhaps can help to answer the questions mentioned above, because only a positive answer can justify the continuation of the therapeutic attempts in diabetes.

PANCREAS TRANSPLANTATION

As shown in the Table 1, according to Sutherland (29,30) several techniques have been used for transplantation of a whole pancreas or of a segment of the organ. Although allograft rejection is the major limiting factor in the use of pancreas transplantation as a therapeutic measure, technical problems have to be solved first.

TABLE 1. Techniques for pancreas transplantation[a]

Type of Transplant	Clinical Cases	Currently Functioning	
		No.	Percent
A. Pancreaticcoduodenal—28 Total			
1. Cutaneous doudenostomy	8	0	0%
2. Roux-en-y doudenojejunostomy	20	0	0%
B. Segmental pancreas—158 Total			
1. Deliberate cutaneous fistula	2	0	0%
2. Ducto-ureterostomy	8	0	0%
3. Duct ligation	12	0	0%
4. Open duct intraperitoneal	17	3	18%
5. Pancreatico-enterostomy	29	4	14%
6. Duct injection with polymers	90	15	17%
Total	186	22	12%

[a] Collection of pancreatic transplantation results at the end of 1981 (From Sutherland, refs. 29, 30, with permission).
[b] Neoprene 29 (3 Fxn), prolamine 27 (5 Fxn), polyisoprene 15 (3 Fxn), silicone rubber 11 (3 Fxn) and cyanoacrylate 8 (1 Fxn).

EXPERIMENTAL STUDIES

From experimental animals, it can be concluded that pancreatic coduodenal transplantation in larger animals was nearly completely unsuccessful because of the enormous technical problems. Segmental pancreatic grafts are simpler to perform. The drainage of the pancreatic liquid is directed either to the jejunum or to the ureter. Duct-ligated grafts as well as duct-obliterated grafts using various liquid synthetic polymers have been used as well as intraperitoneal transplantation of pancreatic segments without duct ligation. The advantage of one or the other method is still under debate. From the endocrinological point of view, transplantation of pancreatic tissue restores plasma glucose of a diabetic animal if more than 20% of the normal pancreatic mass is transplanted (31). However, there is little information regarding the effect on late complications. Only in rats was it shown that transplantation of a whole pancreas can inhibit renal and ophthalmic diabetic lesions.

Almost all pancreatic transplants have been performed with venous drainage of the graft into the iliac vein or vena cava of the recipient. The liver—the major site of insulin degradation—is initially bypassed. This might explain some minor abnormalities in glucose metabolism of such animals. However, it is not determined whether or not they are of importance in the prevention of late complications. In general, experimental pancreas or segmental transplantation has given further encouragement to scientists to try these techniques in humans.

CLINICAL STUDIES

Clinical pancreas transplantation during the last 20 years has passed several stages that cannot all be mentioned here. The most important development is the change from grafting a whole gland to the transplantation of only a segment of the organ. Interestingly, the first pancreas transplant in 1967 was performed as a segmental graft. With this approach, the body and the tail (approximately 50%) of the pancreas is removed and the splenic artery (or celiac axis) and splenic vein (or portal vein) are used for anastomoses to the iliac vessels of the recipient (Fig. 1). Of the many variations, two major techniques should be

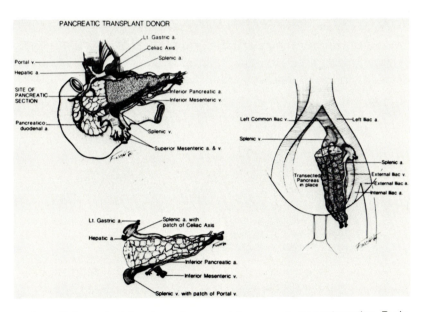

FIG. 1. Schematical drawings of segmental pancreatic transplantation. Body and tail are transplanted with anastomoses of splenic vessels of donor pancreas to iliac vessels of receipent. (From Sutherland, refs. 29, 30, with permission).

discussed, i.e., whether pancreatic duct acclusion or the technique with an open duct is perferable. For both techniques, there are several arguments. Briefly, the American group of Najarian and Sutherland (22) in Minneapolis as well as the British group of Calne in Cambridge are in favor of free drainage, whereas the French group of Dubernard (7) and Traeger in Lyons found duct occlusion with neoprene superior. Because segmental transplantation is now used in many groups in various countries, the definite number of the patients treated in that way is difficult to obtain. According to Sutherland (29,30) and to Dubernard (7) and Traeger, at the end of 1981, the situation was as listed in Table 2. During the last year, evidence has accumulated that kidney transplantation some months prior to pancreas or segmental transplantation is superior to a simultaneous grafting of both organs. The survival time of the pancreas was definitely prolonged when it was transplanted later than the kidney (7). When technical problems did not occur and when rejection was suppressed, carbohydrate metabolism of the grafted patients was found to be normal regarding daily blood glucose measurements, but some patients showed abnormalities, as shown by Sutherland in 1981 (30) in Figs. 2, 3. They were furthermore studied in detail by Pozza (23). He found in patients with segmental pancreatic grafts that the oral glucose tolerance

TABLE 2. *Various modes of pancreas or segmental transplantation*

	References[a]
1. Whole pancreas	
A. Pancreaticoduodenal	
With cutaneous-duodenostomy	[9,14,15]
With Roux-en-Y duodenojejunostomy	[9,12,16–19]
B. With cuff papilla of Vater and	
anastomosis of duct to loop of jejunum	[23,24,24a]
C. En block with other organs	[21,26]
2. Segmental pancreas graft—Body and tail	
A. Duct ligated	[25,32,33,38,40,42]
B. Pancreatic ductoureterostomy	[11,19,27,28]
C. Roux-en-Y pancreaticojejunostomy	[12,19,27,30,31]
D. Duct injected with synthetic polymers	[43–49]
E. Intraperitoneal with duct left open	[36,42,44,50–52]

[a] From Sutherland, ref. 30, with permission.

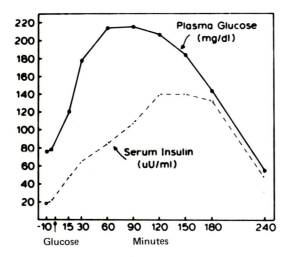

FIG. 2. Glucose tolerance test 1 year after segmental pancreas transplantation to diabetic recipient. (From Sutherland, refs, 29, 30, with permission).

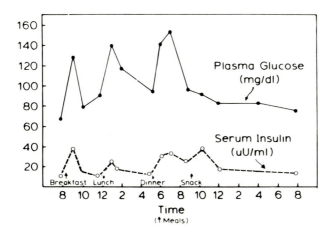

FIG. 3. Metabolic profile 1 year after segmental pancreas transplantation to diabetic recipient. (From Sutherland, refs, 29, 30, with permission).

test and the i.v. GT were abnormal. Similar results were obtained by Largiader et al. (19). Whether this is due to the denervated organ, to damage by neoprene, or to the lack of the surrounding exocrine tissue remains open.

Furthermore, at present, there are still not enough patients with long functioning grafts, and consequently, careful examinations of the retina and the renal function for a definite statement with regard to the effect on late complications cannot be made to form a conclusion. Some anecdotal observations, however, are in favor of this hypothesis, as seen in cases described by Gliedmann et al. (12) and by Sutherland (29,30). They could show by sequential renal biopsies in two patients with a whole pancreatic graft that after several months up to 2 years, a marked improvement of the glomerular lesions had occurred.

Although the overall success rate of pancreas or segmental transplantation is still low, it seems that the technical problems can be overcome. In addition, most of the early patients were nearly moribund from secondary complications when their operations were performed. The survival rate since 1977, when patients in better conditions had transplants, is much higher. At present, the best approach appears to be segmental transplantation with total duct occlusion and intraperitoneal placement to absorb residual secretions. From the results of the four groups with the largest experience, namely, Minneapolis, Lyons, Cambridge, and Stockholm, there is some evidence that pancreas transplantation could be as successful as renal transplantation in patients with renal end-stage failure. This, however, holds only true for those diabetics who already undergo immunosuppression because of a prior renal transplant or in the very few situations where the threatening complications of the disease will be more dangerous for the patient than the hazards of immunosuppression. With disregard of the great problems of immunosuppression at present, pancreas organ transplantation can be summarized as follows:

1. Pancreas (segmental) transplantation most probably does not guarantee perfect metabolic control; the remaining abnormalities can be compared with the situation of latent diabetes.

2. Segmental transplantation is superior to whole organ transplantation.

3. There is evidence that late complications after pancreas transplantation can be prevented or arrested in experimental animals and in patients with long-lasting survival of the graft.

4. Pancreas or segmental grafting should be performed *after* kidney transplantation.

ISLET TRANSPLANTATION

Experimental Data

Although isolated islets have been used for single, experimental *in vitro* and even *in vivo* studies for many years, the technique of enzymatic isolation of the endocine tissue, according to Lacy and Kostianovsky (17), was the basis for the numerous following *in vivo* studies as an alternative to pancreas transplantation. The reason for this is obvious insofar as the transplantation procedure is safer and simpler for the recipient: it can be repeated several times, islet banking should be possible in order to wait for a good match, and manipulations of the islet prior to transplantation possibly could reduce immunogenicity.

About 10 years ago, the first systematic transplantation studies with isolated islets or with dispersed pancreas were started (1,11). In the meantime, a great number of results have been obtained mostly in small animals (rodents), some also in larger animals, and a few in humans. They cannot all be reported here and we refer the reader to the excellent detailed overview given by Sutherland (29,30).

INDUCTION OF DIABETES

Most islet transplant experiments have been performed in animals with chemically induced diabetes or with diabetes following pancreatectomy. Both models are artificial factors to the metabolic changes by the loss of the whole pancreas. Therefore, natural models of animal diabetes such as the ob/ob and db/db mouse have also been used, and moreover diabetes has been induced by infection with the EMC-virus. It has been shown that islet transplantation can reverse diabetes in those models characterized by B-cell destruction and insulin deficiency. This supports the idea that diabetes by chemical B-cell destruction is the most simple method that can be used in order to study the effect of islet transplantation. Undoubtedly, most experiments have been done in rats, especially because of the possibility to use inbred strains; mice, guinea pigs, hamsters have been used, and larger animals such a pigs and dogs very rarely have been used for isolated islet transplantation. One of the main reasons is the difficulty to reach a yield of islets high enough to compensate the diabetic disorder. The source of islet tissue was adult pancreas, neonatal and fetal pancreas.

SITE OF TRANSPLANTATION

Many sites have been used for implantation of isolated islets or of dispersed pancreatic tissue, but the intraportal route or the use of the splenic vein for intrahepatic location have been mostly reported, as well as injection of the islet tissue into the peritoneal cavity. Thus the liver and the spleen are the most favorable sites because the number of islets necessary for compensation of the diabetic state is smaller there than in other anatomical sites (Fig. 4).

METABOLIC EFFECTS

In rats using amounts of 400 to 800 islets from two to three donors, a nearly complete normalization of glucose metabolism can be observed (Table 3). The oral glucose tolerance test—as in animals grafted with a whole pancreas—is not normal, probably due to the denervation and the lack of the cephalic phase of insulin secretion, as shown elegantly by Dr. Renolds' group (32).

ISLET TRANSPLANTATION AND THE EFFECT ON LATE COMPLICATIONS

For a long time, it has been known that in experimental diabetes, renal and other lesions similar to those observed in humans occur after several months. The renal lesions are especially similar to those associated with diabetes in humans. It has been proved that these lesions are not a direct result of the agent-inducing diabetes but are secondary to the abnormal environment to which the kidney is exposed. Kidneys transplanted

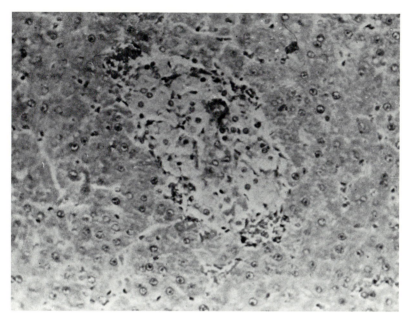

FIG. 4. Syngeneic islet transplantation into the liver via the portal vein. Lodging of the islet within the hepatic tissue without inflammatory reactions 114 days after implantation (HE stain.)

TABLE 3. *Metabolic parameters of normal, diabetic, and transplanted rats at age of 9 months*

	Normals ($N = 9$)	Diabetics	
		No transplant ($N = 20$)	Transplanted ($N = 16$)
Glycosuria (%)	0	>2%	0 n = 11
			>2% n = 5
Urine volume (ml/24h)	10.7 ± 0.7	79.2 ± 23	14.3 ± 36
Fasting−BG (mg/dl)	78.2 ± 11.1	337.3 ± 20.9	76.1 ± 6.3
Fasting−IRI (μU/ml)	39.7 ± 6.3	13.6 ± 1.6	54.7 ± 9.5
k-value (i.v. GTT)	1.51 ± 10.0	0.35 ± 0.04	1.17 ± 0.05
Body weight (g)	416.8 ± 4.3	229.7 ± 5.7	362.0 ± 9.8

[a] From Federlin, refs 9, 10, with permission.

from normal rats into diabetic rats develop lesions identical to those occurring in the diabetic recipient's own kidneys, and conversely lesions in diabetic rat kidneys disappear or fail to progress after transplantation to normal rats (20). The influence of islet transplantation on established renal lesions is shown by an actual decrease of the mesangial matrix material as evident by the disappearance of the PAS + substance and by the disappearance of the immunoglobulin and complement deposits (Figs. 5 to 7). Furthermore, tubular changes are reversed.

Semiquantitative measurements demonstrate the reduction of affected glomeruli, the reduction of the amount of immunoglobulin and complement within the mesangium. In a quantitative evaluation of the percentages of the tissue components, the rewidening of the capillary lumina is the marked result (5) (Table 4). Further studies have shown that the increased proportion of capillary surface and glomerular basement membrane

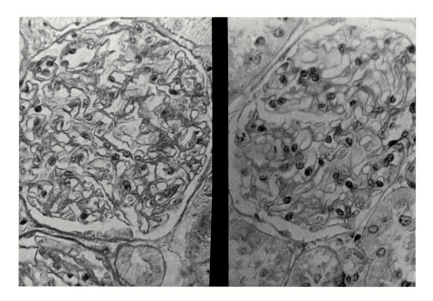

FIG. 5. Influence of islet transplantation upon diabetic renal lesions in streptocotozin-treated rats. **Left:** glomerulus of a diabetic rat 4 months after induction of the disease: slight enlargement of the mesangium with deposition of PAS pos. material. (PAS stain.) **Right:** Same rat 4 months after transplantation of 800 syngeneic islets. Disappearance of the depositions within the mesangial space, normalization of the glomerular structure. (PAS stain)

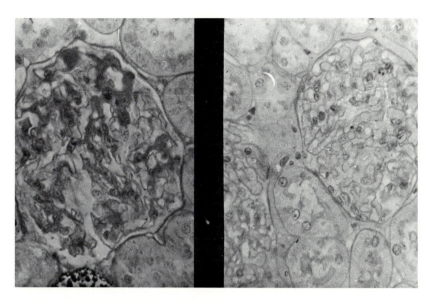

FIG. 6. Influence of islet transplantation upon diabetic renal lesions in streptocotozin-treated rats. **Left:** Glomerulus of a diabetic rat 12 months after induction of diabetes. Massive thickening of the capillaries and enlargement of the mesangial space. (PAS stain.) **Right:** Glomerulus of a rat of the same age; induction of diabetes 12 months previously with islet transplantation following after 4 months. Prevention of diabetic lesions. (PAS stain.)

epithelium interface juxtaposed to the mesangium also declined after transplantation (26). The increase in basement membrane thickness in rats 7 months after induction of diabetes did not decline over a 6-month observation in electron microscopic studies in spite of functional normalization. This might be due to the slow turnover of basement membrane in rats (27).

Furthermore, GLT activity is a good example for glomerular damage and AAP for tubular changes (5) (Fig. 8), as well as Laminin + 7-s collagen, which are further constituents of B.

There are few reports on the effects of islet transplantation on the nerve and eye, but it was clearly demonstrated that rats with transplants do not develop diabetic cataracts and that new vessel formation and retinal capillary dilation do not occur. By ocular fluorometry, it can be shown that islet transplantation reestablishes the integrity of the blood-ocular barrier (15). Also, autonomic diabetic neuropathy was prevented or even reversed (24).

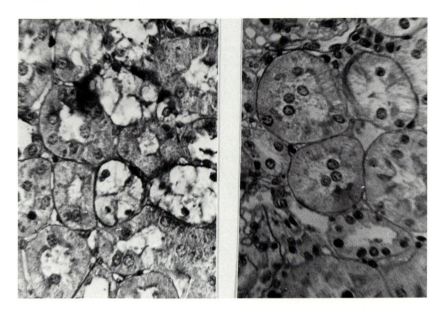

FIG. 7. Influence of islet transplantation upon diabetic renal lesions in streptocotozin-treated rats. **Left:** Tubular cells of a diabetic rat with typical so-called Armanni-Ebstein cells (glycogen-rich cells). **Right:** Prevention of these tubular changes of a diabetic rat by islet transplantation. (PAS stain.)

IMMUNOGENICITY OF ISOLATED ISLETS

Already in the first studies with allogeneic islets, it became clear that this tissue was highly immunogenic. The function of transplanted islets lasted only for a few days. Within the hierarchy of tissue rejection, isolated islets range at the top, even higher than skin, i.e., islets are still more rapidly rejected. Among the many attempts to reduce immunogenicity of islets, the experiments of Lacy and his group (16,17) during the last few years offer substantial hope for further progress in this field. On the basis of the passenger-cell concept in transplantation immunology of Snell (25) and Billingham (2), and stimulated by the successful studies of Lafferty (18) to reduce thyroid immunogenicity by organ culture, Lacy suggested that islet immunogenicity may be mainly caused by transmission of white blood cells within the islet capillaries. In fact, Lacy could demonstrate

TABLE 4. Glomerular components[a]

Age [months]	Group	Capillary walls	Capillary lumina	Mesoangium
2	Normal (N = 3)	7.6 ± 1.1	32.2 ± 1.0	10.2 ± 1.0
5–6	Normal (N = 8)	10.0 ± 0.4	37.0 ± 2.0	17.9 ± 2.3
	Diabetic (3–4 mo) (N = 14)	11.6 ± 1.0	27.3 ± 1.2	28.1 ± 2.1
7–8	Normal (N = 4)	8.9 ± 2.1	30.0 ± 2.8	23.9 ± 2.8
	Diabetic (5–6 mo) (N = 6)	12.7 ± 1.5	26.8 ± 1.1	27.5 ± 4.7
9–10	Normal (N = 7)	10.2 ± 2.1	29.9 ± 1.7	25.2 ± 1.9
	Diabetic(8 mo) (N = 6)	13.5 ± 2.5	23.0 ± 1.1	34.4 ± 2.7
	Transplant (3–4 mo.d.) (N = 8)	11.4 ± 1.2	36.6 ± 2.2[c]	22.7 ± 2.5[b]
11–12	Diabetic (10 mo) (N = 3)	15.3 ± 2.5	19.6 ± 3.3	40.9 ± 7.9
	Transplant (5–6 mo.d.) (N = 4)	8.8 ± 0.8[c]	35.0 ± 2.8	28.9 ± 2.3

[a] Basis 50 glomeruli per rat. Quantiative measurement of the changes within the glomerular structure in diabetic rats after islet transplantation. Transplanted animals show marked decrease of the percentage of the mesangial space and rewidening of the capillary lumina. Reduction of the thickness of capillary walls in transplanted animals after 9–12 months. From Bretzel et al., *unpublished data.*

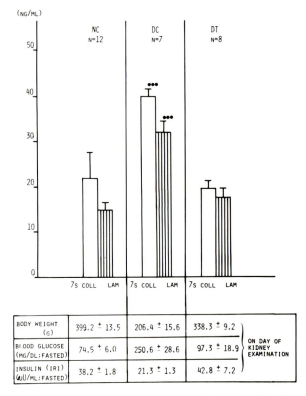

FIG. 8. Serum levels of 7S-collagen and Laminin P2 in diabetic rats, transplanted rats and controls. Note normalization of serum levels in transplanted rats. (From Bretzel et al., *unpublished*)

that cultivation of islet at 24°C prior to transplantation was followed by a marked prolongation of graft survival. With additional use of ASL, islet function in allogeneic recipients was extended from 5 to 7 days to 100 days (17).

Using specific antisera against the Ia-antigens on the surface of lymphocytes (cytotoxic ab) of mice, it was possible to prolong islet function in an allogeneic recipient, crossing a major histocompatibility barrier up to 200 days (9). Furthermore, there is evidence for the fact that very clean islets are not fully immunogenic because animals grafted with such very carefully selected islets remain normoglycemic even without immunosuppression

(Barker, *personal communication*; 10). Thus, some hope has emerged that the immune barrier for transplantation of islets can be lowered, which would have important consequences also for the further research in this field. Another requirement for the use of islets as a treatment of diabetes is preservation in order to collect enough islets or to define the best moment for transplantation with regard to the recipient.

PRESERVATION OF ISLET TISSUE

For short-term preservation as well as for long-term preservation, various methods have been used, namely tissue culture, cold storage, and cryopreservation. Rodent islets can be kept in culture for approximately 1 to 2 weeks before transplantation. However, for longer storage, other techniques are of greater advantage. Cold storage is the simplest way. Several studies have shown that at 4°C rat islets can be successfully transplanted after storage for up to 108 hr (21). The method was less successful in preserving islets derived from larger animals such as dogs. In such experiments, islet transplantation could be successfully performed when the tissue had been stored at 4° for 24 hr but not longer (28).

The most important development has been made using cryopreservation of islet tissue. The endocrine tissue can be stored for many months at 196°C without loss of viability. From many results obtained during the last few years, we would like to show some data of our own laboratory (3,4), which demonstrate no change in glucose stimulated insulin release of cryopreserved islets, whereas insulin biosynthesis was markedly reduced (Fig. 9).

As shown in further studies by Schatz et al. (13), a 2-day culture increases the capacity for biosynthesis up to 50%. Furthermore, the morphology of cryopreserved islets that shows some derangement is nearly normalized after a 7-day culture (Fig. 10). Thus, the prerequisites for islet banking, i.e., preservation of islets from various donors have been already established. There are very few studies with cryopreserved islets from larger animals such as pigs and from human donors with partial success. They have been transplanted in allogeneic recipients.

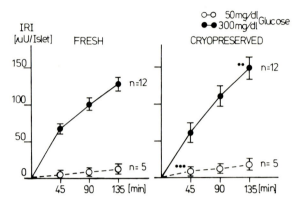

FIG. 9. Insulin release of fresh or cryopreserved rat pancreatic islets. (From Bretzel et al., ref 5, with permission.)

Clinical Data

Although fetal islet tissue offers some advantages because of the limited amounts that are available, adult islets, for ethical reasons, were mostly used in the few attempts of treatment in diabetic patients. Unfortunately, the size of the gland, its architecture, the fibrous tissue, and the fat content make it very difficult to isolate pure islets from human pancreas. From experimental data in dogs, it became evident that purification is not necessary from the endocrinological point of view and that dispersed pancreas may be equally used. For comparison, whereas the yield of pure isolated islets of a human pancreas was about 5% of the total islet mass, the final yield in dispersed tissue from normal cadaver glands reached 60%.

The first allogeneic islet transplantation in humans with dispersed pancreatic tissue was performed in 1977 by the Minneapolis group of Professors Najarian and Sutherland (22) in seven patients. The suspension was given intraportally and intraperitoneally and was tolerated without complications. The success was limited; only half of the patients showed a reduction in the daily insulin requirement. As an explanation, the low number of islets (about 40,000) and possibly the high immunogenicity of the injected material have to be taken into account.

According to the information by Dr. Sutherland, who collects

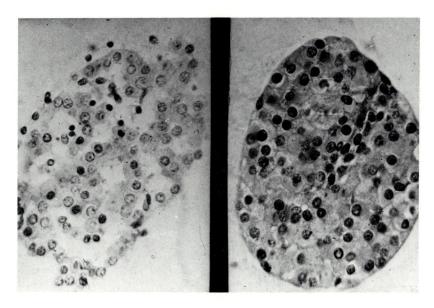

FIG. 10. Left: Islet after thawing after 8 months of cryopreservation. Irregular pattern of islet cells (disarrangement) with open space between islet cells and segregating cells at the periphery. (HE stain.)
Right: Islet after cryopreservation of 8 months and following 14 days culture at 37°C. Normal compact pattern of an islet without signs of damage. (HE stain.)

as far as possible the data of islet transplantations that are not routinely listed in the transplant registry, at the end of 1981, 74 transplantations of islets have been performed in 69 patients. At the end of the year, no functioning graft was reported.

Most of the patients showed a temporary reduction in insulin requirement and a few became temporarily completely free from insulin. The longest survival time was observed in a patient of Largiader's group (14): a female diabetic suffering from the disease for 22 years did not require insulin for nearly 1 year after intrasplenic transplantation of islets from a 2-½ year-old child. In another case, fetal islets were functioning for 11 months in a patient described by Chastan et al. (6), even after a period of cryopreservation, and the patient was also free from insulin for the time mentioned. Thus, in single situations, islet transplantation in humans seems to work, although the exact conditions that permit long survival are not always worked out.

Finally, the present situation in islet transplantation can be described as follows:

1. In experimentally induced diabetes, islet transplantation leads to normoglycemia and, with single exceptions, to aglycosuria. Oral glucose tolerance remains abnormal most probably due to the denervation of the islets.

2. In spite of minor abnormalities of the glucose metabolism, animals with transplants show definitely prevention of late complications at the kidney, eye, and nervous system. Furthermore, early lesions can be reversed. Equal experiences in humans are still lacking.

3. Islet transplantation in humans has been found to be safe, but so far it is a largely unsuccessful method in the treatment of diabetics.

Further research should be concentrated on (a) Increase of the yield of viable islets from donor pancreas, and (b) Reduction of islet immunogenicity as already worked out to some extent in experimental animals.

REFERENCES

1. Ballinger, W. F., and Lacy, P. E. (1972): Transplantation of intact pancreatic islets in rats. *Surgery*, 72:175–186.
2. Billingham, R. E. (1971): The passenger cell concept in transplantation immunology. *Cell. Immunol*, 2:1–12.
3. Bretzel, R. G., Schneider, I., Zekorn, T., and Federlin, K. (1981): Cryopreservation of rat, porcine and human pancreatic islets for transplantation. In: *Islet Isolation, Culture and Cryopreservation,* edited by K. Federlin, R. G. Bretzel, 152–160. Thieme, Stuttgart and New York.
4. Bretzel, R. G., Schneider, J., Zimmermann, I., Küppers, B., Weise, M., and Federlin, K. (1981): Urinary excretion of alanine aminopeptidase and total proteinuria in experimental diabetes mellitus before and after islet transplantation. *Contr. Nephrol.*, 24:153.
5. Bretzel, R. G., Schneider, J., Dobroschke, J., Schwemmle, K., Pfeiffer, E. F., and Federlin, K. (1980): Islet transplantation in experimental diabetes of the rat. VII. Cryopreservation of rat and human islet. Preliminary results. *Horm. Metab. Res.*, 12:274.
6. Chastan, P., Berjon, J. J., Gomez, H., Meunier, J. M., and Doutre, L. P. (1980): Implantation de pancréas foetaux chez un diabétique insulinodépendant. *Nouv. Presse Med.*, 9:353–354.

7. Dubernard, J. M. (1982): Pancreas segmental transplantation under surgical and endocrinological aspects. Workshop of the EASD-study group on Artificial Insulin Delivery Systems and Pancreas-Islet Transplantation. IGLS Austria, February 1–2, 1982.
8. Faustman, D., Hauptfeld, V., Davie, I. M., Lacy, P. E., and Schrefler, D. C. (1980): Murine pancreatic B-cells express H-2K and H-2D but not Ia antigens. *J. Exp. Med.*, 151:1563–1568.
9. Faustmann, D. (1981): Preliminary report. *Diabetes Outlook*, 16: 1–3.
10. Federlin, K., Bretzel, R. G., and Weise, M. (1981): Reversion of nephropathy in experimental diabetes by islet transplantation. In: *New Approaches to Insulin Therapy*, edited by K. Irsigler, K. N. Kunz, D. R. Owens, H. Regal, p. 389–403. MTP Press Limited, Lancaster.
11. Federlin, K. Helmke, K., Slijepcevic, M., and Pfeiffer, E. F. (1973): Transplantation of isolated islets of Langerhans into pancreatectomized rats. *Diabetologia*, 9:66.
12. Gliedman, M. L., Tellis, A., Soberman, R., Rifkin, H., and Veith, F. J. (1978): Long-term effects of pancreatic transplant function in patients with advanced juvenile-onset diabetes. *Diabetes Care* 1:1.
13. Gonnermann, B., Schatz, H., Schäfer-Spiegel, R., Schneider, J., and Federlin, K. (1981): Insulin biosynthesis and release of cryopreserved rat islets. In: *Islet Isolation, Culture and Cryopreservation*, edited by K. Federlin, R. G. Bretzel, pp. 161–164. Thieme, Stuttgart and New York.
14. Kolb, E., and Largiader, F. (1981): Transplantation of pancreatic microfragments in patients with juvenile diabetes. In: *Islet Isolation, Culture and Cryopreservation*, edited by K. Federlin, and R. G. Bretzel, p. 188 Thieme, Stuttgart and London.
15. Krupin, T., Waltman, S. R., Scharp, D. W., Oestrich, C., Feldman, S., Becker, D., Dallinger, W. F., and Lacy, P. E. (1979): Ocular fluorophotometry in experimental diabetes mellitus: the effect of pancreatic islets isografts. *Invest. Opthalmol. Vis. Sci.*, 18:1185–1190.
16. Lacy, P. E., and Kostianovsky, M. (1967): Methods for the isolation of intact islets of Langerhans from the rat pancreas. *Diabetes*, 16:35.
17. Lacy, P. E., Davie, J. M., and Finke, E. H.: Prolongation of islet allografts survival following in vitro culture (24°C) and a single injection of ALS. *Science*, 204:312.
18. Lafferty, K., Cooley, M., Woolnough, J., and Walker, K. (1975): Thyroid allograft immunogenicity is reduced after a period in organ culture. *Science*, 188:259.
19. Largiader, F., Baumgartner, D., Uhlschmid, G., and Binswanger, V. (1982): Pankreas- und Nierentransplantation bei diabetischer Nephropathie. *Dtsch. Med. Wochenschr.*, 107:527–530.
20. Lee, C. S., Mauer, S. M., Brown, D. M., Sutherland, D. E. R., Michael, A. E., and Najarian, J. S. (1974): Renal transplantation in diabetes mellitus in rats. *J. Exp. Med.*, 139:793–800.
21. Matas, A. J., Sutherland, D. E. R., Payne, W. D., and Najarian, J. S. (1978): Transplantation of neonatal rat islet tissue after in situ and cold ischemia. *Diabetes (Suppl. 2)* 27:440.
22. Najarian, J. S., Sutherland, D. E. R., Matas, A. J., Steffes, M. W., Simmons, R. L., and Goetz, F. C. (1977): Human islet transplantation: A preliminary report. *Transpl. Proc.*, 1:233.

23. Pozza, G. (1982): Discussion remark. 1. Workshop Meeting of the EASD-Study Group on Artificial Insulin Delivery Systems and Pancreas-Islet Tranplantation. IGLS, February, 1–2, 1982.
24. Schmidt, R. E., Nelson, J. S., and Johnson, E. M., Jr. (1981): Experimental diabetic autonomic neuropathy. *Am. J. Pathol.*, 103:210–250.
25. Snell, G. B. (1957): The homograft reaction. *Am. Rev. Microbiol.*, 2:439–458.
26. Steffes, M. W., Brown, D. M., Basgen, J. M., and Mauer, S. M. (1980): Amelioration of mesangial volume and suface alteration following islet transplantation in rats. *Diabetes*, 29:509–515.
27. Steffes, M. W., Brown, D. M., Basgen, J. M., and Mauer, S. M. (1979): Glomerular basement membrane thickness following islet transplantation in the diabetic rat. *Lab. Invest.*, 41:116–118.
28. Sutherland, D. E. R., Kretschmer, G. J., Matas, A. J., and Najarian, J. S. (1977): Experience with auto and allotransplantation of pancreatic fragments to the spleen of totally pancreatectomized dogs. *Trans. Am. Soc. Artif. Intern. Organs*, 23:723–725.
29. Sutherland, D. E. R. (1981): Pancreas-islet transplantation. *Surgical Rounds*, July.
30. Sutherland, D. E. R. (1981): Pancreas and islet transplantation. *Diabetologia*, 20:161, 435.
31. Toledo-Pereya, L. H., Castellanos, J., Manifacio, G., and Lillehei, R. C. (1979): Basic requirements of pancreatic mass for transplantation. *Arch. Surg.*, 114:1058–1062.
32. Trimble, E. R., Siegel, E. G., Ghinovci, A., Renolds, A. E. (1980): The importance of early insulin responses in oral glucose tolerance: studies in islet-transplanted and normal rats. *Diabetologia* 19:320 (Abstract), 380.

Afterword

Rachmiel Levine

City of Hope Medical Center, Duarte, California

When I remember the energetic and brash young man whom I met 25 years ago in Frankfurt, I cannot believe that he, Ernst Pfeiffer, is 60 years, and that I'm even older. But when I scan over his curriculum vitae and bibliography, the honors received, the multiplicity of his activities, then I must conclude that he began publishing on his first birthday. Otherwise, it does not seem possible.

Let me confess that in 1957, it was not Ernst Pfeiffers' sound work that attracted me, but the fact that he was a young man who argued with me; he had no respect for his elders. He debated very strongly and at length. This I appreciated very much. Respectability kills a good scientist's initiative.

I have been told by Professor Federlin that I should make a resume. This would be impossible. In this volume are many excellent reports and articles. It is not possible to do justice to the work and the people involved in a few pages. The reader should consider my remarks simply as the impressions of an interested scientist.

In the 46 years that I have been in this field, I have seen a tremendous transformation. Diabetology in 1936 centered around organ physiology and intermediary metabolism: the precise significance of the D:N ratio, overproduction versus underutilization, mechanisms of ketosis, etc. We have come a long way since then. You have heard today the attempts to integrate the techniques and outlook of molecular biology into our field of medicine. This is, of course, going on in many other fields. Professor Czech discusses the present status of the molecular biology of insulin receptors and its meaning in the transduction of the insulin message. I am not going to discuss which is more important, the hormone or its receptors. They are both important. As a matter of fact, I can make a good argument that neither the hormone nor the receptor are as important as the "mediator" since it leads to the postreceptor events, i.e., the hub of metabolism. We also heard another exposition in an area—let me call it geographical molecular biology—by the great artist in the field of diabetology, the Matisse of our field, Dr. Lelio Orci. Not only does he explore the intimate geography of the cell, but he does it very satisfactorily and most esthetically.

Very early in his scientific life Professor Grodsky became interested in insulin secretion when very few researchers were involved with it. He presented his data and theories about synthesis and secretion, as to which batch of insulin comes out first. We thought that after 2 or 3 years, he would exhaust the subject. He hasn't. He keeps on uncovering new and important aspects of the subject.

I was very glad to listen to an old friend about an ever new subject. Werner Creutzfeldt reviewed in masterly fashion the relation of gastrointestinal hormones to the functions of the endocrine pancreas. The subject has been with us for years, ever since 1908, but more intensively in recent years. His review demonstrated that we may now be able to construct a meaningful neuroendocrine pathway between the GI tract and the endocrine pancreas. It is not purely hormonal; it has neurological elements to it. Some of the problems with transplantation of the whole pancreas might be due to interruption of the neuroendocrine pathways.

Hans Ditschuneit brought out certain aspects of the behavior of the somatomedines, NSILA, etc., which seem to me of great importance, not only in regard to possible relations between NSILA and atherosclerosis, but also the relationship of NSILA to the origin and etiology of type II diabetes. This is a very intriguing concept.

I was delighted to hear the clear exposition by Dr. Gepts, whose name is synonymous with the histology of the diabetic pancreas. He clarified the present status of the ultrastructure of the gland as seen in the two major types of diabetes. I was especially interested in his stressing the possible increase in the number of PP cells. Even the viruses came in for a paper. The viruses are intriguing as well in the etiology of type I diabetes. It formed an excellent review of the present situation.

An old subject, the sulfonylureas, is undergoing a scientific revival. Interesting differences are being revealed between the first and second generation of sulfonylureas, even though these do not yet explain why sulfonylureas continue to control the hyperglycemia despite a lessening of their effect on insulin secretion.

Most interesting to me is the possibility that the open-loop system might provide a hint as to whether chronic hyperglycemia itself causes the microvascular complications. I was delighted to hear Kerner's review of the artificial pancreas and the pump. The advantages of the pumps and also the gaps in our understanding that still exist were carefully delineated.

The review by Professor Federlin on transplantation was an excellent summary of his own work and that of others. It brings with it the hope that using Lacy's techniques, especially that of removing the passenger lymphocytes, plus cryopreservation, might spare us the problem of transplanting a complete and complex organ. The possibility of preventing the rejection of the endocrine portion of the organ would be a real advance in therapy.

I should like to conclude by thanking the contributors to this volume for a delightful and intellectually stimulating symposium. It is indeed a rich feast in honor of a most deserving worker in our field.

Subject Index

Subject Index

Acarbose
  action, 156
  supplementary therapy, in insulin-dependent diabetics, 156
A cells
  distribution, in maturity-onset diabetes, 95,97
  gap junctions, 17,21
  in juvenile-onset diabetes, 99–102
  quantitative changes, in mouse pancreas, in diabetes, 117
Acetyl choline, 27
Acromegaly, 71
  IGF levels in, 78–79
Adipocyte
  biological effects of insulin and IGF receptors in, 48–49
  IGF binding, 84
  interaction of insulin and IGF receptors in, 49
  isolated, biological action of IGF Ulm in, 79–80
Adrenalin, levels, in insulin-induced hypoglycemia, 173,178
Amino acid, concentrations, effect of glucose control, 195–196
Amylase
  pancreatic, 27
  salivary, 27
Amyloidosis, islet, in maturity-onset diabetes, 96–97
Antidiabetics, oral, 135
  interaction with other drugs, 146–147
  and vascular complications, 152–155
Arginine, infusion
  effect on glucagon level, 194–195
  effect on growth hormone level, 192,194
Arteriosclerosis, in diabetes, 157
  and oral antidiabetics, 152–155
Atherosclerosis
  insulin-like activity in, 69
  pathogenesis, insulin-like growth factors in, 70–71,77,91
Atropine, effect, on insulin response, 56
Autoimmunity
  cell-mediated, and insulitis, 104–105
  in chronic glomerulonephritis, early research, 4–5
  in pathogenesis of diabetes, 121–123

B cells
  changes, in maturity-onset diabetes, 97–98
  chemical destruction, 105, 211–213
  damage
    viruses causing, 113
    in juvenile-onset diabetes, 102–106
  distribution
    in maturity-onset diabetes, 95,97
    in mouse pancreas, in diabetes, 117,120
  functional deficiency, in maturity-onset diabetes, 98
  gap junctions, 18,20,21–23
  insulin compartments, size, 32–33,38

231

B cells *(contd.)*
  insulin processing, prediction, 33–34
  insulin secretion, regulation by glucose, 27–40
  in juvenile-onset diabetes, 99–101
  quantitative changes, in juvenile-onset diabetes, 101–102
  secretory mechanism, 36–38
  sensitivity, changes, in sulfonylurea therapy, 147
Beta cells, *see* B cells
Biguanides
  contraindications, 155
  side effects, 155–156
Biostator, 6,59,140–143,190
Buformin, 148,155

Carbutamide, 129
Cataracts, diabetic, and islet transplantation, 215
Catecholamines, levels, effect of blood glucose control, 195
CCK, *see* Cholecystokinin
Cell
  coupling
    electrical, 21
    intercellular, 18
    metabolic, 21–23
  proliferation
    blood-borne growth factors in, 70
    effect of insulin and IGF receptors, 48–49,51
    role of IGFs, 43,77
    role of insulin, 43
    serum factors with insulin-like activity in, 70
Chlorpropamide, 137
Cholecystokinin
  as insulin releaser, 58–59,66
  as neurotransmitter, 58,66
Cholesterol, blood level, effect of blood glucose control, 196–197
7S-Collagen, serum levels, effect of islet transplantation, 215,218

Coma diabeticum, *see* Diabetic coma
Cortisol, level
  effect of blood glucose control, 192,194–195
  in insulin-induced hypoglycemia, 173,178
Coxsackie B virus, and diabetes, 112–116,118
C-peptide, 144–145,148
Cryopreservation, of islet tissue, 219–221
Cytomegalovirus, and diabetes, 111–112

D cells
  distribution, in maturity-onset diabetes, 95
  gap junctions, 18,23
  in juvenile-onset diabetes, 99–102
  quantitative changes, in mouse pancreas, in diabetes, 117
Diabetes, 64
  age at onset, and insulinitis, 107–108
  atherosclerosis in, insulin-like activity and growth hormone levels in, 71
  IGF levels in, 78–79
  induction, 211–212
  juvenile-onset (type I), 93,98
    pancreatic morphopathology in, 98–106
    pathogenesis, 130
    therapy
      ideal, 181
      patient's role in, 181
      urine testing in, 181–183
  maturity-onset (type II), 93
    pancreatic pathomorphology, 94
    pathogenesis, 130
    response to glibenclamide therapy, 143–144
    treatment objectives, 130, 156–157

SUBJECT INDEX

and obesity, 130,148
oral therapy, drug interactions in, 146–147; *see also* Antidiabetics, oral
pathogenesis, insulitis in, 121–123
primary, 93
secondary, 93
spontaneous, in guinea pig, 118
treatment, with oral hypoglycemic agents, 129–163; *see also* Insulin
types requiring insulin therapy, 169
vascular complications
  effect of blood glucose control, 198
  and oral antidiabetics, 152–155
  pathogenesis, 189
  prevention, 180–181
and virus, *see* Virus
Diabetic coma
  low-dose insulin therapy, 167
  mortality, decrease in, 165–166
Diabetology, 227–229
Diabur 5000, 181–183
DNA
  replication, effect of insulin and IGF receptors, 48–49,51
  synthesis, role of IGF I in, 77, 80–82
Dopamine, stimulation, by biosynthetic human insulin, 181
Dye, injection, in study of cell communication, 22

Electrophysiology, in study of cell communication, 22
Encephalomyelitis, Venezuelan equine, and diabetes, 118
Encephalomyocarditis virus (EMC-virus)
  and diabetes, 113–115, 116–117,119–120
  diabetes induction with, 211

diabetogenic subtypes, 117–122
Endocrine cell, monolayer culture, heterogeneous clusters, 21–22
Enteroinsular axis, 56
Enteropancreatic axis, effect of glibenclamide, 148
Exercise, effect on growth hormone level, 192–193

Fat cell, *see* Adipocyte
Fetal calf serum, biological action, 80,82–83
Fibroblast, IGF binding, 84,90
Foot and mouth disease virus, and diabetes, 112,118
Free fatty acid, levels
  effects of blood glucose control, 196–197
  effects of insulin therapy, 173,175
  response to exercise, 193,196

Gap junction
  in islet cell communication, 18–25
  modulation, according to cell function, 23
  morphological demonstration, 21–23
Gastric inhibitory polypeptide
  discovery, 59
  incretin activity, 59–61,64–65
  release, 59,66
    amino acid-induced, 58
    in chronic pancreatitis with steatorrhea, 62–63
    feedback control, by insulin, 59,66
    by HC1, incretin effect, 58
Gastrin, in insulin secretion, 58
GIP, *see* Gastric inhibitory polypeptide
Glibenclamide, 133
  action, 134–137
    on insulin receptors, 148

SUBJECT INDEX

Glibenclamide, 133 (contd.)
  blood sugar curve produced by, 140–143
  effect on platelets, 154
  extrapancreatic effects, in obese diabetics, 148
  for secondary failure during first-generation sulfonyl-urea therapy, 137–140
  stabilization achieved with, time course, 147
  therapy, combined with insulin, 149
  in treatment of obese, maturity-onset diabetics, 148–150, 156
  vascular effects, 154
Glibornuride, blood sugar curve produced by, 140,141
Glicaride, effect on platelets, 154
Gliclazide
  action, 134–137
  blood sugar profile produced by, 140,142
  effect on platelets, 154
Glipizide, 137,140
  blood sugar profile produced by, 140,142
Gliquidone, blood sugar profile produced by, 140,143
Glomeruli, lesions
  effect of islet transplantation, 214–218
  and pancreatic transplantation, 210
Glomerulonephritis, studies of, 4
Glucagon
  cells
    distribution, 11–19
    in juvenile-onset diabetes, 99
  level
    effect of glucose control on, 192–195
    in insulin-induced hypoglycemia, 173,177
    in response to arginine infusion, 194–195
Glucoquant, 183–185

Glucose
  assimilation, in glibenclamide therapy, 143,144
  blood
    changes, in low-dose insulin therapy, 167–168
    control
      effects on counterregulatory hormone levels, 191–195
      effects on diabetic microvascular complications, 198
      effects on metabolite levels, 195–197
      in prevention of vascular complications, 180–181
    determination by artificial pancreas, 140–143
    effect of i.v. injection of secretin and glucose, 61
    in excretory pancreatic insufficiency, 62
    in insulin-induced hypoglycemia, 173,174
    normalization, 189–191
    in pathogenesis of diabetic microvascular complications, 189
    profile produced by sulfonylureas, 140–143
    response to exercise, 193
    testing, 182–185
  effect, on insulin secretion and specific activity, 34–36
  metabolism
    after islet transplantation, 212–213
    after pancreatic transplantation, 208–210
  potentiation
    by glibenclamide, 145
    by sulfonylureas, 137–140
  urinary, estimation, 181–183
Gonadotropin, 27
Growth hormone
  and atherosclerosis, 71
  level, effect of glucose control on, 191–192

secretion, in insulin-induced
    hypoglycemia, 173,176–179

Haemoglukotest 20-800, 183–184
Hepatoma cells, H-35, insulin and
    IGF receptors in, 49
Hexokinase
    blood glucose estimation with,
        183–184
    urinary glucose estimation with,
        182
Hexose, transport activity, effect of
    insulin and IGF II receptors
    on, 48,50–51
Hormone, *see also specific hormone*
    counterregulatory
        effect of improved glucose
            control on, 191–195
        in insulin-induced
            hypoglycemia, 173–180
    gastrointestinal
        interaction, effect on islet
            function, 65–66
        and islet function, 55–68
Hyalinosis, islet, in maturity-onset
    diabetes, 96–97
beta-Hydroxybutyric acid, blood
    levels
    after insulin treatment, 173–180
    in low-dose insulin therapy,
        167–168
Hypoglycemia
    insulin-induced, secretion of
        counterregulatory hormones
        after, 173–180
    from oral diabetes therapy,
        symptoms, 147
    prevention, GIP in, 59
    in response to glibenclamide, 146
Hypophysectomy, IGF levels after,
    78–79

Immunosuppression, and pancreatic
    transplantation, 210
Incretin, 55–56
    activity, of gut extract, 64–65
    definition, 55
    unknown, 65,66
Incretin effect, 56
Influenza, and diabetes, 111
Insulin
    action, 41–42,47–49,80,82
        on cell proliferation, 43
        IGFs as mediators, 43
    artificial delivery systems,
        190–191
    blood level, in secretory
        pancreatic insufficiency, 62
    cells, distribution, 11–15
    competitive binding with IGF,
        83–87
    Des-Phe, 170–174
    discovery, 165
    displacement of IGF binding,
        83–87
    effect, on IGF II receptor,
        49–50
    human
        action, vs. porcine insulins,
            171–173
        biosynthetic
            action, 173–176
            studies of, 180
    labeling, 28–29
    marking, 27
        critical period, 37–38
        glucose concentration during,
            34–36,38
    membrane effector system, and
        biological effects, 41–42
    newly synthesized
        preferential secretion, 27–39
        storage, 29–31,38
    porcine
        action, 173–176
        conversion to human insulin,
            171
    preferential secretion, effects of
        secretagogues, 36
    preparation, by recombinant
        DNA techniques, 171
    preparations, 169–170
    purification, 28–29
    purified, 169–170

Insulin *(contd.)*
  receptors, 41
    affinity purification, 43–44
    antibodies, 44
    binding kinetics, 47
    cross-reactivity, with insulin-like growth factor receptors, 42
    effect of glibenclamide, 148
    effect of growth, 84–87
    homology, with receptors for insulin-like growth factors, 41
    immunoprecipitation, 44
    subunit structure, 44–46,51
    tissue distribution, 47–48
  secretion
    effect of gastrin-CCK family, 58–59
    effect of i.v. injection of secretin and glucose, 61
    enhanced by GIP, 58
    in glibenclamide therapy, 143–144
    in juvenile-onset diabetes, 101–102
    potentiation by sulfonylureas with glucose, 137–139
    rigidity, 130–131
    stimulation
      by drugs, 132–147
      effect on B-cell gap junctions, 23–24
      by glibenclamide plus glucose, 145
      by secretin *in vitro*, 56–58
  specific activity
    calculation, 28
    effect of glucose concentration during marking period, 34–36
    ratio, 36
    secreted vs. cellular, 30–33
  vs. sulfonylureas, for diabetes treatment, 149–153
  therapy, for diabetes, 165–188
    closed-loop system, 185–186
    individualization, 181
    low-dose, 167–169
    with sulfonylureas, 149
    supplemented with acarbose, 156
Insulin infusion pump, 190,
    portable, 191
Insulin-like activity, 69
  atypical, 69–70
  nonsuppressible, 69–70
  serum fractions, 70–71, biological activity, 71–76
Insulin-like growth factor
  I
    biological activity, 77
    identity with somatomedin C, 77
    isolation, 73
    membrane signaling system, 41–42
    receptor, 41
      affinity labeling, 44
      binding kinetics, 47
      biological actions, 48–49
      similarity to insulin receptor, 45
      subunit structure, 45–46,51
      tissue distribution, 47–48
    similarity to proinsulin, 76–77
  II
    isolation, 73
    membrane signaling system, 41–42
    receptor, 41
      affinity for IGF II, effect of insulin on, 50–51
      affinity labeling, 44
      binding kinetics, 47
      biological action, 48–49
      response to insulin, 49–50
      structure, 46–47
      tissue distribution, 47–48
    similarity to proinsuliln, 76–77
  interrelationship with atherosclerosis, 70–71
  receptor
    on cell surface of cultivated smooth muscle cells, 83–88
    effect of growth on, 84–87

serum level, radioimmunoassay, 88,89
Ulm
 biological activity
  compared to IGF Zurich, 79–83
  in isolated fat cells, 79–80
  in smooth muscle cells, 79–83
 purification, 77–78
 specific activity, 79–80
Insulitis, 102–103,115,121–125
 and age at onset of diabetes, 103–104
 in animals, 105
 biphasic course, 123–125
 etiology, 104–105
 frequency, in juvenile-onset diabetes, 103
 rodenticide-induced, 105
Islet cells
 antibodies, appearance, in onset of diabetes, 103
 communication, 18–25
 distribution, 11–18
 necrosis, in virus infection, 115–117
 quantitative changes, in juvenile-onset diabetes, 101–102
Islets of Langerhans
 appearance
  in juvenile-onset diabetes, 98–101
  in maturity-onset diabetes, 94–95
 cells, see Islet cells
 cellular composition, in maturity-onset diabetes, 97
 fibrosis, in maturity-onset diabetes, 95
 hyperactive, in juvenile-onset diabetes, 99,100
 incubation, 28
 inflammation, see Insulitis
 insufficiency, 117,121
 isolated, immunogenicity, 216–219
 isolation, 28
 lymphocytic infiltration, in juvenile-onset diabetes, 102–103
 mouse, changes in, in virus infection, 116–117,120
 pseudoatrophic, in juvenile-onset diabetes, 98–99,105
 structure
  distortion, in juvenile-onset diabetes, 102
  regulatory influences of, 11–26
 tissue
  banking, 219
  cold storage, 219
  cryopreservation, 219–221
  culture, 219
  preservation, 219–221
  volume changes, in maturity-onset diabetes, 94
 transplantation, 205,211–222
  clinical data, 220–222
  experimental data, 211
  and late diabetic complications, 212–218
  metabolic effects, 212–218
  site, 212–218
  survival times, 220–222

Ketoacidosis, diabetic, 165–166
 insulin resistance in, 169
 treatment, 166–169
Kidney
 lesions, effect of islet transplantation on, 212–216
 transplantation, and pancreas transplantation, 208,211

Lactic acidosis, side effect of oral antidiabetics, 155,157
Lactogen, placental, 27
Laminin, serum levels, effect of islet transplantation, 215,218
Lipid, blood levels, effects of blood glucose control, 196–198
Liver, plasma membrane, IGF binding, 84

SUBJECT INDEX

Lymphocyte, transfer experiments, to transfer diabetes, 123–124

Measles, and diabetes, 111
Metabolites, concentrations, effect of blood glucose control on, 195–197
Metformin, lactic acidosis caused by, 156–157
Microtubule, disruption, effect on insulin secretion, 36–38
Mononucleosis, infectious, and diabetes, 112
Mumps, and diabetes, 112,118
Muscle, effects of insulin and IGF receptors in, 48–49

Nephropathy, diabetic
  effect of blood glucose control on, 198
  and pancreas transplantation, 215
Neuropathy, diabetic
  effect of blood glucose control, 200
  and islet transplantation, 217
Nexus, see Gap junction

Obesity, and diabetes, 130,148
Optisulin, see Insulin, Des-Phe
Osmolarity, changes, in low-dose insulin therapy, 167,169

Pancreas
  annular, 16,18–19
  artificial endocrine, 190–191
    blood sugar determination by, 140–143
    early history, 6
    in study of GIP-cell responsiveness to insulin, 59–61
  embryonic development, and heterogeneity of islets, 16–19
  exocrine, insufficiency, 61–64
  gross changes
    in juvenile-onset diabetes, 98
    in maturity-onset diabetes, 94
  head, posterior lobe, 16–18
  human, sampling regions, 16–17
  lymphocytic infiltration, phases, 123,125
  mouse, pathomorphology, in diabetes, 116,120
  monolayer culture, cell communication study, 21
  pathomorphology, in diabetes, 93–110,115
  rat, sampling regions, 13
  transplantation, 205–211
    in animals, 206–207
    clinical studies, 207–211
    techniques, 205–208
Pancreatic polypeptide cells
  distribution, 11–19
  in juvenile-onset diabetes, 98, 100–102
Pancreatitis, chronic, incretion effect in, 61–62
Pancretin, effect, on GIP release and insulin response, 63
Parabiosis, 4
Parathyroid hormone, 27
Pentamidine, insulitis induced by, 105
Pfeiffer, Ernst, 1–9,225
Phenformin, 151,155
Platelets, effects of oral antidiabetics on, 154
Poliomyelitis, and diabetes, 111
Preproinsulin, 30
Proinsulin
  conversion to insulin, 29–31
    stoichiometry, 30–32,38
  displacement of IGF binding, 83–84
  labeling, 28–29
  newly synthesized, storage, 29–31,38
  processing, 29–31
  purification, 28–29
  similarity to IGF, 76–77

Prolactin, 27
  secretion, in insulin-induced hypoglycemia, 175–180
Protein, synthesis, stimulation, by IGF, 77,80,82

Reflectometers, 182–183
Reovirus type 1, and diabetes, 121
Retinopathy, diabetic
  effect of blood glucose control, 198
  and pancreas transplantation, 210
RNA, synthesis, role of IGF in, 77, 80–82
Rubella, and diabetes, 112–113,110

Secretin, 56–58,65
Secretory granule, insulin marking in, 27,36–38
Smooth muscle,
  cultured cells
    activity of IGF Ulm in, 79–83
    demonstration of IGF receptors on cell surface of, 83–88
    transport of amino acids into, effect of IGF on, 80–83
  growth promotion, by sera from patients, 77–79
Somatomedin, 70–71
Somatomedin C, identity with IGF I, 77
Somatostatin
  cells
    distribution, 11–16
    in juvenile-onset diabetes, 99
  paracrine effects, 64,66
Sulfamidopiridine, derivatives, 133
Sulfonamide, derivatives, 133
  action, 133–134
  dosages, 133

Sulfonylurea, 129
  derivatives, 133–134
  effects, in obese diabetics, 131–132
  first generation, 134–140
  vs. insulin, for diabetes treatment, 149–153
  second generation, 134
  thyrostatic action, 155
  vascular effects, 154
Synalbumin, 69–70

Tetragastrin, in insulin secretion, 58
Thyroglobulin, 27
Thyroid hormone, secretion, and sulfonylureas, 155
Tolbutamide, 133,137,139
  and vascular complications of diabetes, 152
Triglyceride, blood level, effect of blood glucose control on, 196–197

Varicella virus, and diabetes, 112
Vasoactive intestinal peptide (VIP), 64,66
Vasopressin, 27
Virus, see also specific virus
  B-cell damage from, 104–105
  and diabetes, 111–128
    in animals, 116–117
    in humans, 111–116
  potentially causing diabetes, 111–113
  subtypes, in diabetogenesis, 117–122

Weight, see also Obesity
  reduction, in treatment of diabetes, 130–132,156